D0403577

LIFELINES

Living Longer, Growing Frail,
Taking Heart

Muriel R. Gillick, M.D.

W · W · NORTON & COMPANY
NEW YORK · LONDON

Lines from the poem "Sailing to Byzantium" by W. B. Yeats reprinted in the United
States with the permission of Scribner, a Division of Simon & Schuster from
The Collected Poems of W. B. Yeats, Revised Second Edition, edited by Richard J.
Finneran. Copyright 1928 by Macmillan Publishing Company; copyright renewed
© 1956 by Georgie Yeats; reprinted throughout the world (excluding the United
States) with the permission of A. P. Watt Ltd. on behalf of Michael B. Yeats.

For information about permission to reproduce selections from this book,
write to Permissions, W. W. Norton & Company, Inc.,
500 Fifth Avenue, New York, NY 10110

The text of this book is composed in Adobe Garamond with the display set in Eden
Composition by Molly Heron
Manufacturing by Maple-Vail Book Manufacturing Group
Book design by Rubina Yeh

Library of Congress Cataloging-in-Publication Data

Gillick, Muriel R., 1951–
Lifelines : living longer, growing frail, taking heart / by Muriel R. Gillick.
p. cm.
Includes bibliographical references.
ISBN 0-393-05002-5
1. Frail elderly—United States. 2. Frail elderly—United States—Case studies.
3. Aging. I. Title.
HQ1064.U5 G475 2000
305.26'0973—dc21   00-033941

W. W. Norton & Company, Inc., 500 Fifth Avenue, New York, N.Y. 10110
www.wwnorton.com

W. W. Norton & Company Ltd., 10 Coptic Street, London WC1A 1PU

1 2 3 4 5 6 7 8 9 0

To my parents, Ilse and Hans Garfunkel,
in the hope that they continue to keep frailty at bay.

CONTENTS

INTRODUCTION

Frailty in Our Time

Throughout the developed world, people are living far longer than they used to. Life expectancy at birth in the United States is now seventy-four years for males and seventy-eight years for females. A man who has made it to age sixty-five without succumbing to congenital conditions (the bane of infancy), homicide or motor vehicle accidents (the threats in young adulthood), or heart disease or stroke (the major killers in middle adulthood) can anticipate living another fifteen years. A woman who reaches sixty-five can expect to live another twenty years. Are those extra years a time to look forward to? Have the improvements in public health, diet, and medicine that extended our lives also improved the quality of those years? Or can we expect a long period of disability, chronic illness, and dependence before death?

Specialists in aging have hotly debated whether medicine has ushered in a new era characterized by the "compression of

morbidity": a long, robust old age that is followed by a brief period of decline and then death.[1] Studies in the 1980s made it
painfully clear that while some people remained spry into their
late eighties and nineties, many endured a prolonged period of
failing health and progressive disability before the end of their
lives.[2] The years from sixty-five to eighty, on average, were a time
of vigor, but after eighty the likelihood of a gradual and difficult
decline was very great. Most people who made it to their eighties
or nineties suffered from the elusive condition known as *frailty*.

What exactly is frailty? The crux of frailty is impairment in
multiple domains leading to profound difficulty functioning in
daily life.[3] Typically, frailty involves suffering from limited
reserves: the frail person is always on the edge of a precipice, with
barely enough organ capacity to get by. A slight breeze can knock
the frail individual over; the common cold may trigger a worsening of emphysema; a low-grade fever may precipitate heart failure; a urinary tract infection can lead to incontinence.

Precisely because frailty usually stems from a mix of problems,
there is no antifrailty pill on the horizon, no wonder drug that
will simultaneously fix eyesight, restore hearing, and repair joints.
Although frailty cannot be cured and can only sometimes be prevented, a great deal can be done to improve the lives of the frail:
hope rather than despair should be the response to this widespread condition. Preventing frailty in those who are not afflicted
and ameliorating it in those who are is one of the greatest challenges facing our generation.

In 1997, for the first time, epidemiologists found evidence of
a fall in the percentage of individuals facing a protracted period
of disability in old age.[4] While this is encouraging news, the reality is that nearly two-thirds of women and almost half of men
over the age of eighty-five either need extensive assistance in their
everyday activities to remain at home or are already living in a
nursing home.[5] Although the proportion of older people who are

frail has fallen, the growing number of very old people will translate into *increasing* absolute numbers of frail people in the coming decades. Moreover, frailty is not a condition that older people experience for a matter of months. Typically, once frailty sets in, it lasts for several years. There is no solid data on the average duration of frailty, and a minority of people are impaired only transiently, after an acute illness, for instance, but the majority can anticipate from three to five years, and sometimes as long as ten or fifteen years, in a state of frailty.[6]

This book is about the *experience* of the frail elderly, the lives of all those who struggle to find comfort, well-being, and meaning in the last months or years of life. Few poems are written about them and seldom do magazine articles praise their courage or their contributions to mankind. The vigorous elderly are the media idols—those who stay strong and independent well into old age and then have the fortune to die rapidly, with little fuss. Bookstore shelves are replete with manuals purporting to teach us how to stay robust into old age. Those who are dying are also the subject of a growing number of books and newspaper articles. The frail, by contrast, are ignored even though frailty currently affects 6.5 million people over age sixty-five, and by the year 2020 it will affect more than 10 million people. For those over age eighty-five, it is commonplace.[7]

My professional life is devoted almost exclusively to the frail elderly. Most of my patients have multiple disabling physical problems, cognitive decline, or both. I take care of this population because I find it tremendously rewarding and challenging. But I also find that both patients and their families are often ill-equipped to handle the decisions that face them when frailty develops. Over and over, I try to guide them through the new terrain they must traverse—I discuss with them whether they should undergo particular surgical procedures, what supports they need to survive, in what kind of environment they should live. I also find that most people have little experience in dealing with chronic illness—they are accustomed to medical problems that develop rapidly, are treated swiftly, and get better. What I try to help them understand is that the approach to problems in the case of frailty is different. The goal is seldom cure but rather amelioration: fixing the one component of frailty that is amenable to treatment, making life tolerable by addressing concomitant emotional problems, or enabling the individual to compensate for his deficits by means of homemakers and home health aides. I have also come to believe that the critical determinant of quality of life among the frail is often the spiritual rather than the medical dimension of existence. Discovering meaning in life, a purpose, a connection to other individuals and other generations, makes dependence and disability bearable. This kind of spiritual need is at least as important among the elderly as it is in younger age groups, where it is the basis for the search for community and the renewed interest in religion.

Lifelines seeks to help the frail elderly and their families cope with their condition by describing some of the most common causes of frailty and discussing the medical, ethical, and social issues they engender. I believe these issues are best addressed concretely, by rooting the discussion in real cases. I have therefore chosen to weave each chapter around the stories of four people drawn from my clinical experience: Jack Simon, a dynamic, self-made man who was catapulted into frailty by a stroke; Ben Frank, a soft-spoken widower who slid into frailty as one organ system after another began to fail; Catherine Endicott, who moved stepwise into frailty with each of several heart attacks; and Leyla Keribar, who endured Parkinson's disease but became frail when she developed dementia on top of her physical condition. In each instance, the patient is a composite, based on several real individuals, but with a single person at the core. Through these clinical tales, I hope to develop an approach to assessing, treating, and living with frailty that makes sense for the majority of people.

Because frailty is not a single disease, but rather a condition that by definition arises from the interaction of multiple problems, there are many points of entry into frailty. Just as there are many ways of becoming frail, there are many paths a person may follow once he or she has become frail. Each person typically confronts a variety of difficult issues in the course of struggling to cope with frailty. Foremost in my mind as a physician are the physical issues. Patients who are frail learn that the goal of their medical care is not and cannot be to cure them of the multitude of medical problems that make them frail. Rather, the goal of care is usually to maximize their function, to promote their independence and well-being by controlling their incontinence or improving their heart failure. Sometimes, one of the many problems that jointly render them frail can be definitively repaired: Jack Simon had a cataract that was removed, resulting not only in better vision but also in a dramatic change in his ability to care for himself; Leyla Keribar had a hip joint replaced, ending a cycle of pain and progressive loss of mobility even though her Parkinson's disease continued to take its toll.

Often, frail elderly people develop a critical illness that forces them to make difficult decisions about the scope and type of medical treatment to undergo. They and their families need to decide whether to submit to what are often extremely unpleasant technological interventions in exchange for what is often only a small chance of survival. If they do undergo maximal treatment and do survive, they are frequently left with even more debility and dependence than they had prior to the acute illness. Each of the four people in this book faced such decisions and each chose a different approach. Ben Frank unequivocally aimed for life-prolongation, whatever the physical and emotional cost. Leyla

Keribar's family felt her quality of life was such that they wanted her to be spared all treatments except those devoted to her comfort. Jack Simon chose a course midway between these extremes, opting for an intermediate level of treatment, which entailed accepting potentially curative treatment but not the most aggressive treatments available so as to reduce the chance of further disability. Catherine Endicott initially favored whatever medical technology had to offer, but over time, as she became increasingly frail, gradually modified her position.

Physical problems represent only one of the many challenges facing the frail and their families. At least as important as the pills they take and the hospitalizations they endure is the environment in which they live. Frail older people often find it difficult to remain in the home where they have resided for many years. If they do stay home, they may need to renovate the house so that it is equipped with assistive devices such as grab bars or a raised toilet seat. They need a panoply of home services to help with shopping, cleaning, and cooking, and sometimes bathing and dressing. Painful as the decision is to move into a new home, often located in a new community, sometimes hundreds of miles away from their roots, it is often essential. If the surrounding neighborhood has changed in character and their friends have died or moved away, a transition to a new environment may be very desirable. Fortunately, there are now many different living arrangements conducive to the needs of frail older people. Ben Frank managed to remain in the two-bedroom apartment where he had lived for sixty years and had raised his two children, but he needed to accept considerable outside help. Leyla Keribar moved in with her daughter and son-in-law until she was so frail that she needed the round-the-clock supervision provided by a nursing home. Jack Simon moved into a continuing-care retirement community, together with his wife. Catherine Endicott moved out of the three-family house where she had grown up and then had cared for her ailing husband to live first in an apartment and then in an assisted-living complex. In each case involving a move, the transition was initially traumatic but ultimately a relief to all concerned.

Frailty presents emotional as well as physical problems. Adjusting to a state of at least partial dependence is commonly very painful, especially in a society that places a premium on self-reliance. The cowboy and the self-made man are American icons, not the elder with a walker who maintains his dignity in the face of assaults on his bodily integrity. The caricature of the older person as crotchety and impatient reflects the reality that depending on others for help with bathing or dressing or cooking can engender frustration. Waiting for assistance, asking for help, and being confronted daily with one's deficits tries the equanimity of even the most easygoing individual.

Coping with frailty may trigger depression, which happened with Ben Frank. He had never before been depressed, although he had had quite a bit of experience with this condition since his wife had suffered from recurrent depression for many years. Normally a cheerful and not terribly demanding man, Ben was profoundly saddened by his wife's death. He managed to keep on going, learning to use a microwave, eating almost daily at the corner delicatessen, and his spirits improved as he realized he was not helpless. He was pleasantly surprised to discover that the many household activities for which his wife had always been responsible were not beyond his grasp, even at age eighty. Slowly, he began to shape a new life for himself, spending time with a small circle of friends, going out to clubs and restaurants that his wife would have disdained. His newfound self-sufficiency necessitated a freely functioning body and an intact mind. When his body began to betray him—when he became so short of breath with exertion that he could no longer walk to the corner store, when his hearing became so impaired that he had trouble communicating with his friends—he became depressed. A combination of medical treatment to improve his heart failure, a hearing aid, and resolution of his depression enabled him to deal with his increasing frailty.

For Catherine Endicott, loss of independence created a devastating sense of anxiety. This proud, capable woman who had lived alone for more than twenty years after the untimely death of her husband at age fifty-seven, and who had supported her family financially for the seventeen years of his disability, was suddenly terrified of being alone. She telephoned her daughters constantly, and made several middle-of-the-night trips to the hospital emergency room. The major intervention that enabled her to stay out of a nursing home for several years was a move into assisted living. Just knowing that help was immediately available vastly decreased her anxiety level. She slept at night instead of tossing fitfully in bed. Socializing with other residents took the edge off her daytime anxiety.

Frailty became an overwhelming problem for Leyla Keribar when she developed mild dementia on top of her physical ailments. She had adjusted to using a walker to compensate for her difficulties with balance. She was reconciled to giving up some of her social activities because of her mobility problems. She had accepted that she was no longer the helper in the family but instead needed help with shopping and cooking and housework. But when she began developing memory problems and difficulty expressing herself, when she began losing her way, she panicked. Her self-esteem was intimately bound with her sense of control over her life. Once she could no longer trust her mind to work, she felt a helplessness she had not experienced when only her legs were undependable. Her fears escalated to the point where she wanted someone with her at all times. Eventually, her family could not handle her constant calling out, her endless neediness, and they moved her to a nursing home.

Frailty has implications for physical health, for mental health, for where one lives, and also for spiritual well-being. Maintaining relationships, contributing to society at large, earning an income, raising children, and numerous other activities give meaning to people's lives. Frailty jeopardizes a person's capacity to engage in those pursuits that make his or her life worth living. Simply slowing down and having to devote hours every day to personal hygiene and to one's health—taking pills, going to doctors, using assistive devices for bathing and walking—limits the amount of time available for other things. Difficulties with mobility, with hearing, with vision, often put a damper on efforts to continue the work and play that previously afforded satisfaction. For the final months or years of life to be meaningful, the frail older person needs either to adapt his previous activities to accommodate his health status or to find new paths to spiritual fulfillment and new creative outlets. Retaining a sense of worth despite one's disabilities in a society that tends to disparage the impaired older individual is probably the most daunting challenge of frailty.

Every person who becomes frail and each family that discovers frailty in its midst faces a perilous journey. The questions of where to live and what medical interventions to accept will come up over and over again. The struggle to cope with frailty both emotionally and spiritually—to avoid anxiety and despair on the one hand, and to find peace and satisfaction on the other—will mark each journey. There is no one answer for everyone. This book will look at the journeys of four very different people in the hope that readers will identify with many of their dilemmas: their stories—how they made decisions to limit medical treatment, how they coped emotionally, where they lived, how they found meaning in life—are offered in an effort to help guide the way for the millions who are frail, their families, and their friends.

LIFELINES

CHAPTER 1

The Roads to Frailty

When Louis Pasteur established beyond a reasonable doubt that microorganisms cause disease, medicine was transformed. What had been a murky realm of miasmas and vapors became an orderly world of cocci and bacilli. Whereas previously a single "condition" could be associated with different symptoms in different sufferers, now a given "disease" implied an invariant set of symptoms. Sicknesses such as pneumonia or tuberculosis or endocarditis metamorphosed into very specific entities: each was caused by a particular germ, which produced a predictable series of changes in the human host it invaded. The discovery of antibiotics—chemicals that killed germs, thereby curing disease—was the crowning achievement of the germ theory revolution. Not only was the germ theory a powerful way of explaining disease, of understanding causality and pathogenesis, it was also a means to effecting a cure.

3

The idea that bacteria are responsible for much of human disease, while initially dismissed as preposterous, proved so powerful and compelling that the temptation has been to view *all* human illness in the same reductionist light.[1] We would like to find a single cause for each disease, including coronary artery disease, cancer, and Alzheimer's disease—hence the excitement surrounding high cholesterol and oncogenes and familial forms of dementia. While these disorders do not appear to be caused by an infectious agent, the hope is that they may nonetheless prove to be due to a single potentially correctable abnormality, whether environmental or genetic. Because the germ theory of disease has been so successful in its realm, and treatment of chronic diseases such as rheumatoid arthritis and diabetes has been less dramatically effective, patients and physicians find explanations of disease that involve multiple factors far less intellectually satisfactory than the unifactorial causes invoked for infections.

If diseases that are due to multiple interacting factors are viewed with suspicion, much more puzzling is the disorder known as frailty. At least coronary artery disease is a single entity, whether it develops primarily from high blood pressure, high cholesterol, cigarette smoking, genetic predisposition, or a combination of several of these. Symptomatic treatment is identical, regardless of the pathway leading to the disease. But frailty is a different kind of entity. People who are frail are dependent in several activities of daily living—basic aspects of life such as bathing, dressing, and walking. Several of their organ systems operate with marginal reserves, each of which is at risk of catastrophic failure. Because the systems involved in generating frailty are typically interlinked, deterioration in one sphere usually precipitates a cascade of adverse effects. But because there are many combinations of problems that produce frailty, it is a far more heterogeneous condition than coronary artery disease.

Frailty takes many forms and can be reached by many roads. Understanding the kinds of journeys that people take to reach frailty is helpful because the journey is sometimes more easily recognized than the destination itself. Individual patients are only seldom given the label "frail" by their physicians, though epidemiologists and geriatricians use this categorization all the time in studying groups of people. Nursing home residents are frail; community-dwelling elders who require long-term care are frail; people over eighty-five exhibit a very high rate of frailty. But because the diagnosis is rarely made explicit, it is useful to become familiar with the paths that lead to frailty. If you recognize the path, you can see where it is heading, and you will not be surprised when you arrive.

For most people, the road to frailty is a long, winding highway along which they make several stopovers. After each stop, they are a little more dependent, a little more impaired, than they were before.[2] Usually they develop discrete problems along the route, problems that make them more fragile. The person with arthritis, for example, may develop macular degeneration and then diabetes, three entirely separate difficulties that attack different bodily functions. One causes problems with mobility, one with vision, and one might lead to recurrent hypoglycemic attacks (episodes of feeling faint from low blood sugar, usually due to excessive medication). Sometimes people have a single chronic disease that produces frailty because it affects many distinct parts of the body. For example, multiple sclerosis, over time, can cause problems with walking, difficulty with urination, and trouble thinking. A single disease such as cancer can gradually cause symptoms in multiple domains: metastases to bone are typically painful; metastases to the back may produce spinal cord compression and paralysis; and metastases to the brain can cause seizures or confusion.

In some instances, individuals do not follow a road, but instead stray from the road, only to fall off a cliff. They are vigorous one day and frail the next.[3] The most dramatic example is stroke, or, as it has been dubbed, "a brain attack." A blood clot chokes off the circulation to part of the brain, or, alternatively, bleeding occurs in the substance of the brain, irreversibly destroying tissue. Or a previously asymptomatic person might suddenly have a massive heart attack, leaving him with so much heart damage that he can no longer do many of the daily chores he always took for granted. Even after extensive rehabilitation, both the individual with a stroke and his counterpart with a heart attack may find themselves very limited in their activities.

Still other people become frail not from their physical problems alone but because they have emotional or cognitive problems on top of their bodily malfunctions. The same degree of arthritis and hearing loss and emphysema that is eminently tolerable in one person may present insurmountable difficulties to someone else who has a lifelong history of manic-depressive disorder. The combination of visual loss and heart disease that necessitates taking a few pills and having a part-time housekeeper might be catastrophic if the individual develops even mild symptoms of Alzheimer's disease.

There are many roads to frailty. The best way to come to grips with the landscape and learn to recognize the destination before arrival is by following the travels of real people as they journey toward frailty.

Ben Frank

The telephone rang just as my family finished dinner. It was my old college friend Susan, calling from New York. We spoke a few times a year and saw each other from time to time. I knew she wouldn't call me long distance unless there was a problem.

"It's my father," she blurted out. "He's in the hospital." I remembered Susan's father: he was a dignified, quiet man. I remembered him together with Susan's mother, a sharp-witted, domineering woman who did almost all the talking. On the rare occasions when Ben had gotten a few words in during a conversation, he proved to have a dry sense of humor. I had not seen him in ages, though I knew he had waited on his wife hand and foot for a decade while she suffered from a series of debilitating ailments. I vaguely recalled she had had low back pain and depression. She had died just a year before. During the ten years of her illness he had remained strong and healthy; now that she was gone and he had a chance to enjoy his life, it was evidently his turn to be sick.

"He fell on the floor and couldn't get up. He was on the floor for twelve hours. My brother called him on the phone a couple of times, and when he didn't answer, he got worried. Finally he drove over to investigate and found him just lying there."

"Does he remember falling? Did he actually pass out?"

Susan said he had gotten up from the kitchen table, felt dizzy, and fallen down. He claimed he had never lost consciousness. She added, "I wish he had passed out. It must have been awful to be stuck on the floor like that, helpless. He couldn't get up. He couldn't reach the phone. He tried calling 'Help, help,' but of course nobody heard him."

"So what did they find in the hospital?"

"Nothing much. The doctor said he had a touch of congestive heart failure. His ankles were swollen. So he put him on a medication to get the fluid out of his ankles and now they're going to send him home. I don't see what the fluid had to do with falling."

"I assume they did other tests as well—looking for a heart attack or an irregular heart rhythm?"

"Yeah, they did all that. All negative."

We talked a little about congestive heart failure (CHF), a condition in which the pump function of the heart is impaired, resulting in fluid backing up into places it does not belong—the lungs, the liver, the ankles. Many older people develop congestive heart failure after a heart attack; some are prone to congestive failure because the heart muscle has stiffened from years of elevated blood pressure. Heart failure is often a more serious condition than the average person appreciates: the six-year survival from CHF is less than 25 percent, a considerably more ominous prognosis than for many forms of cancer.[4] On the brighter side, there are several effective medications for CHF that help keep people out of the hospital and also decrease their mortality. In addition to the old standbys, digoxin and diuretics (fluid pills such as furosemide or hydrochlorothiazide), we now have several other classes of drugs that are helpful, such as the angiotensin converting enzyme (ACE) inhibitors and, in some situations, beta-blockers.

Susan was anxious. Her father had never been sick before. He never even got colds, or the flu. The only time she recalled his having seen a doctor was when he had had a collision with the refrigerator and managed to crack a rib. He had been miserable for a couple of weeks, sore but not really sick. He had trouble with his hearing, but Susan felt that did not count as a significant medical problem. He had never had a condition for which he saw a doctor on a regular basis. He had never before taken pills.

Was congestive heart failure just a minor inconvenience, something he would take in stride, or would it significantly affect Ben Frank's life? How would he respond to being diagnosed as having a chronic disease? Would he adjust to taking medication every day, even when he felt fine, or would he deny there was anything wrong and be noncompliant?

I was as concerned about the falls as I was about the CHF. I wasn't convinced from what Susan told me that they were related. Falls can be a devilish problem. They can cause serious damage—Ben had been lucky that he hadn't broken a hip when he hit the floor, and that he was discovered before he developed dehydration or skin breakdown. Not only are falls objectively dangerous, but they can also wreak havoc by creating a terror of future falls in their victims. Some of my patients are so fearful of falling that they do not go outside, and in certain cases rarely even get out of a chair. Pinning down the cause of falls can be tricky as well. Occasionally falls have a single, straightforward cause—low blood pressure, for example. More often, falls are multifactorial—they arise from a combination of factors, such as poor vision (from macular degeneration) plus impaired judgment (from Alzheimer's disease) added to balance problems (from Parkinson's disease).[5] In a handful of cases, no explanation can be established.

Susan was initially not very worried about the fall, perhaps because she assumed it was a onetime occurrence. But when she called again a mere two months later to tell me about the second fall, she was decidedly worried.

The second time Ben Frank fell and couldn't get up, he was wearing a Life Line buzzer. He actually remembered to use it, summoning help by pressing a button when he inexplicably found himself lying on the floor. Within half an hour the response center at the local hospital had gone through all the mandated steps: First, they tried telephoning Ben to make sure the call was not a false alarm, but of course he couldn't reach the phone. Next, they called a neighbor to check on Ben, but the neighbor was out. Finally, they sent an ambulance, broke open the door, and picked Ben up off the floor. He seemed all right to the paramedics, but, just to be sure, they brought him to the emergency room. From then on it was a replay of his first visit. He had an electrocardiogram that was unrevealing. His physical exam provided no clue. This time there was one difference: his serum sodium, the concentration of salt in his blood, was abnormally low. The low sodium was almost undoubtedly due to the diuretic he was taking to reduce the swelling in his ankles.

Whether or not the low sodium was the exclusive cause of the fall, it was probably a contributing factor. A low sodium level can cause confusion as well as balance problems and, in extreme cases, seizures. Ben Frank was admitted to the hospital, and treated by putting his diuretic on hold and regulating his intake of salt and water. He had a variety of other tests which looked for either an alternative explanation for the fall or an alternative explanation for the low sodium. Those tests were all negative, and on the fourth hospital day, Ben went home.

"So, if he doesn't take a diuretic, he goes into congestive heart failure and falls down. If he takes the diuretic, his sodium drops and he falls down. Is he just going to fall all the time?" Susan asked.

We reviewed his other medications. Sometimes it's possible to avoid using diuretics altogether, preventing CHF with ACE inhibitors, for example. Susan studied the labels on her father's medications. He was now supposed to take the heart medication lisinopril, which was an ACE inhibitor, plus digoxin to strengthen his heart. He was scheduled to have a blood test to measure the digoxin level in his blood and to check his sodium.

A week later, Susan called to check in. Having the test done had actually been surprisingly easy—a visiting nurse had come to the apartment and drawn the blood—but the test had disclosed a new problem. Now Ben's potassium was dangerously high. If it went any higher, his doctor told him reassuringly, he would have a cardiac arrest. The good news was that the culprit was almost undoubtedly the new medication, lisinopril. It would have to go.

Since he had to take something or he would again fill up with fluid, his doctor prescribed isosorbide, a vasodilator.

"So, what side effects does this isosorbide stuff have?" Susan wanted to know.

"Well, it can cause headaches," I began cautiously.

"And?" Susan pressed me, sensing my reluctance to continue.

"It can cause dizziness. Nitrates such as isosorbide dilate blood vessels, so blood pools in the veins. That tends to make blood pressure fall, so when you get up, sometimes you feel faint."

"Wonderful! Dad felt faint *before* he took any isosorbide. Now what do I do? Do I call his doctor and tell him I investigated the medication he prescribed for my father and concluded he chose a real loser?"

I was in an awkward position. First of all, isosorbide was not a poor choice, under the circumstances. There was simply no medication without potential adverse effects. Either Ben Frank was singularly unlucky, or the difficulty finding the right combination of medicines was a clue that his system was a bit more fragile than anyone had thought. Second, I was in some respects in a better position to call Ben's doctor than his daughter was, but I wanted very much to remain in the role of interpreter of medical events. I obviously could not try to serve as a consultant to someone I had not seen in five years. We tried to find a way for Susan to express her concern without appearing meddlesome. The compromise we reached was that Susan would be in touch with her father's visiting nurse, she would remind her of Ben's history of dizzy spells and falls, and she would express anxiety about the new medication. The nurse agreed that her patient needed close monitoring and came to his apartment to check his blood pressure the following day.

Ben Frank's blood pressure was perfect when he sat, relaxed, in his living room. When he stood up, it plummeted. Surprisingly, he did not report any dizziness, perhaps because he got up so slowly and so seldom. Ben had been spending most of his time just sitting. He sat and read the newspaper. He sat and watched the news on television. He commented that he even sat when he urinated, since he felt more secure that way. In his quiet, unobtrusive way, Ben was slowing down.

The visiting nurse went into action as soon as she checked Ben's blood pressure. She called Ben's doctor and discussed the situation with him. He, in turn, phoned in two new prescriptions to a nearby pharmacy. The new regimen—a beta-blocker to slow the heart rate and decrease cardiac work, plus hydralazine, a different type of vasodilator from the ill-fated isosorbide—*had* to work.

Three days after he began the new combination of medications, Ben Frank was back in the local hospital emergency room. He could hardly breathe. He assumed the heart failure was back, this time with a vengeance. He had noticed, however, that he had not gained any weight and that his ankles were not the slightest bit swollen. The young intern in the emergency room quickly resolved the paradox: Ben was not in heart failure—he had asthma.

Ben Frank had never before experienced asthma. He had smoked a package of cigarettes a day for fifty years, but thought he had survived unscathed. He was mistaken. Very gradually, imperceptibly, he had developed emphysema. It was mild, so mild that he was asymptomatic until he began taking beta-blockers. The drug caused just enough narrowing of the airways that were already abnormal from emphysematous changes that, for the first time in his eighty-one years, Ben Frank experienced the frightening, suffocating sensation of an acute asthma attack.

Once in the emergency room, a quick examination of his lungs revealed the classic wheezing of asthma. Ben was treated with bronchodilators, medicine that he breathed in through a special mask. An hour later he had improved markedly—but he was nevertheless admitted to the hospital for observation and to make certain he did not relapse. It was his third hospitalization in six months. He went home with yet another set of medications—back on a diuretic, though this time a milder medicine that his doctor hoped would not interfere with his blood chemistries.

Susan saw the preceding months as a series of medical misadventures. She rationalized that her father had always been a very fortunate man, at least in terms of his health, and that it was simply his turn for a measure of bad luck. I saw the situation differently: his new medical problem, congestive heart failure, had *unmasked* several other problem areas that had been lurking below the surface. Taking the medications for his heart first unmasked a kidney abnormality—if his kidneys had been working perfectly, he would most likely not have developed first the low sodium and then the high potassium. Yet another heart medication had revealed his impaired lung function. And the congestive heart failure, the disorder that had triggered his other difficulties, was itself of far greater concern than Ben realized. He had had an echocardiogram, a special test involving bouncing sound waves off the heart to measure how well it pumped. The test showed that every time his heart contracted, instead of pushing out two-thirds of the blood it contained, it expelled only about one-quarter of the blood. It was working at less than half of its normal capacity. Ben Frank was a sick man, and the sickness translated into significant limitations in his ability to do things for himself.

Ben had never been a tremendously sociable person, so when he started going out only once a week, just to the corner store for essentials, instead of two or three times a week, the change was not dramatic. When he started getting up later and going to bed earlier, plus taking a mid-afternoon nap, he did not have to cancel any social engagements to accommodate his new schedule. When he began requiring an hour to get washed and shaved in the morning, instead of his customary fifteen minutes, there was no one around to notice. But all these changes, which Susan was shocked to discover when she spent a weekend with her father, were telltale signs of his slide into frailty.

Catherine Endicott

Catherine Endicott knew all about sickness. For seventeen years she had been the primary caregiver for her husband, who at age forty had been paralyzed by a stroke. One day he had been a moderately successful businessman. The next day he was an invalid. After two weeks in the hospital and a month of intensive rehabilitation, he returned home. He never set foot in his office again.

The Endicotts lived on the second story of a triple-decker house that Catherine's father had purchased for a song. Her mother lived on the first floor and one of her sisters on the third. When Maurice Endicott could no longer work, Catherine found herself a job to support the family. She left her husband alone during the day, with precise instructions for her mother and sister about how many times to check in on him and what to make him for lunch. Sandwiched in between relatives, Catherine felt he was reasonably secure. She was in charge of evenings and weekends. For seventeen years she rarely left the house except to work and to run errands. There weren't many hours left in the day after she finished her paid employment, and she wanted to spend every one of them with Maurice.

The stroke was only the beginning. The same atherosclerotic

process that had fatefully narrowed a major blood vessel in his brain also affected vessels in his heart, producing angina, and affected the circulation to his legs, causing cramps when he took the few steps he was able to manage. The blood vessels to his kidneys were narrowed as well, resulting in the progressive renal failure that ultimately killed him. Catherine nursed him through it all, bringing him his medications, phoning the doctor to report his latest symptoms, and, near the end, when he was bedridden, bringing him meals in bed. In the interim, she had helped him bathe, dress, and shave. She knew all about low-cholesterol diets for heart problems and low-protein diets for kidney trouble. She was so familiar with Maurice's symptoms that she diagnosed her sister's angina well before her sister's physician did.

When, twenty years after her husband died, Catherine developed chest pain, she was certain she had indigestion. She prescribed antacids for herself and persuaded herself that they made her feel a little better. Catherine got chest pain every time she climbed the stairs to the second-story apartment where she still lived, but she blamed the pain on the snack she ate in the late afternoon to tide her over until dinner. She got chest pain while out for a walk with her daughter, which she promptly attributed to a pulled muscle. Her daughter Andrea was skeptical, especially since Catherine could not recall any musculoskeletal injury. She insisted that her mother make a doctor's appointment. Catherine felt she had kept her end of the bargain when she scheduled an appointment for the following month.

In desperation, Catherine's younger daughter, Jennifer, resorted to subterfuge. She persuaded her mother to let her take her shopping. As soon as she had her mother in the car, she drove to the nearest hospital emergency room. Catherine was furious, which promptly gave her chest pain, which, in her daughter's eyes, clearly justified the hijacking. After three hours in the emergency room, she was admitted to the coronary care unit (CCU) with a diagnosis of unstable angina.

Only when she was put on a medical regimen remarkably similar to the one her husband had been on, and finally stayed pain-free for a whole day, did Catherine Endicott admit that her daughters and her doctors were right. She suffered from a narrowing of the blood vessels to her heart, just as Maurice had. Most of the time she felt fine, but when she exercised, her heart required extra oxygen. That, in turn, meant she needed to pump more blood to her heart. The blood vessels were too narrow; she couldn't boost the supply to meet the increased demand, and she experienced pain in the chest. The new medications—three different prescriptions plus an aspirin to thin her blood—functioned in differing ways to allow her heart to work less hard while still getting its job done. As long as her heart worked below a critical threshold, Catherine had no pain.

As soon as she was discharged, Catherine resumed all her usual activities. She went back to her part-time job as a bookkeeper—the same work that had sustained her during the long years of her husband's invalidism. She resumed her second part-time job, as president of the local senior center. She was responsible for organizing trips, for recruiting speakers, and for supervising the other officers, particularly the treasurer, who needed a great deal of supervision. Whenever their schedules permitted, Catherine's two daughters and their husbands came over for Sunday night dinner. Sometimes the grandchildren came along as well. Catherine's mother, in failing health but still alert and living independently, joined them. Cooking for eight every Sunday became Catherine's third part-time job. The shopping alone took several hours: she insisted on fresh fruit from the fruit market, meat from the butcher's, wine from the wine shop, and, if she did not have the energy to bake herself, dessert from the bakery. Since the main course was typically a turkey or a roast, she needed another half-day for the cooking.

Catherine Endicott's fourth part-time job was caring for her mother. She was grateful to her for having helped her look after Maurice in the years following his stroke. She was delighted that her mother had let her live rent-free on the second floor of her triple-decker. Now Catherine had the opportunity to repay her mother for all she had done for her. Every morning she helped her get washed and dressed and they ate breakfast together. In the evenings, Catherine prepared supper for her mother and helped her get ready for bed. They spent the evenings together—two widows, mother and daughter, two friends—reading, watching television, or playing Scrabble. Catherine had never had a social life outside her family, so she did not feel she was missing anything.

For two years, Catherine managed her four jobs. She was irreplaceable at the office, her mother thrived, the senior center grew, and her children delighted in their weekly dinners. Then, just after her seventy-fifth birthday, the chest pain came back.

The pain hit her with all the force of a well-pitched hardball, but she was not wearing a catcher's glove. This time there was no procrastinating, no rationalizing about indigestion or pulled muscles. Catherine could hardly breathe. When the ambulance came to bring her to the hospital, she was pale and clammy, gasping for breath and in severe pain. This time she had a full-blown heart attack.

Catherine found herself in the local hospital CCU, with oxygen piped into her nose, medications dripping into her veins, and all kinds of catheters threaded into assorted blood vessels. She had a Swan-Ganz catheter, a special intravenous passed through the heart and into the blood vessels of the lungs to measure pressures that reflected how well her heart was pumping. She had an arterial line, a catheter in the artery of her wrist, to provide constant measures of her blood pressure. This was necessary because the medication she was on for her heart tended to cause low blood pressure. Catherine was in a cubicle all to herself, but she could hear the relentless beeping of monitoring machines in the adjoining cubicles, each occupied by a heart attack victim.

The first night she was in the CCU, an alarm went off and suddenly three nurses dashed over to the man in the bed to Catherine's left. Moments later, a stream of physicians poured in, equipment was moved into the room, and Catherine heard a frenzy of activity. For twenty minutes there were shouted instructions, messengers darted out with samples of blood, reams of EKG paper trailed outside the opening to the cubicle. Then all was quiet. The man in the next bed had sustained a cardiac arrest: every effort was made to revive him, but the attempts had failed. He died, a man who, she later learned, was ten years her junior, and who had had a heart attack much like hers. Catherine had never been so exquisitely aware of her own mortality.[6]

Catherine Endicott survived, and her physicians recommended that she consider bypass surgery. Unless she did more than merely take medication, she was likely to have another heart attack, and she might well not survive the next one. Catherine summoned her two daughters to her bedside. She collected statistics from the cardiac surgeon and requested a second opinion from another surgeon. She asked for her daughters' recommendations and those of her sons-in-law. Then she announced her decision: she would take her chances with medication.

Andrea and Jennifer were appalled. They argued, they cajoled, but their mother was resolute. They told her she might as well commit suicide rather than wait for the internal time bomb to go off at some unspecified date. Catherine was firm.

"It's my body and I'm not going to put myself through the ordeal of open heart surgery. At my age and with my blood vessels, I have a good chance of having a stroke. That's what the doctors told me. I'd rather die of another heart attack than be reduced to being an invalid by a stroke. I *know* what a stroke is like," she reminded her daughters. "Your father lived for seventeen years after his stroke. To me, it would be a living hell."

"But Dad didn't see it that way," Jennifer ventured.

"I'm not Dad," Catherine snapped. "Besides, he had me to take care of him."

Jennifer cringed at the implicit suggestion that she and her sister would be unable to provide for their mother what Catherine had given their father. "But don't you think that if he had had to make the decision you're faced with, before he got sick, he might also have thought a stroke would be devastating, but after it actually happened, he would learn to live with it?"

"You can learn to live with anything, I suppose, if you have to," Catherine answered. "If you don't have a choice. But I *do* have a choice. Right now I can take care of myself and lead a normal life. I don't want to risk losing my independence tomorrow by having a major operation. If anything changes—I suppose I could start getting chest pain all the time—I'll have to reconsider."

The subject was closed. Catherine Endicott was discharged from the hospital with five different heart medications. She kept a schedule posted on her refrigerator door to help her remember to take all her pills. She tried going back to her part-time jobs, but she found she no longer had the requisite stamina. She did not get chest pain, and she did not even become short of breath, but she was gripped by fatigue, a fatigue so overwhelming that she sometimes had to lie down to rest even before finishing her supper.

The bookkeeping job was the first to go. Her boss, who had

prevented her from retiring when she reached sixty-five and did not really want to let her quit now, suggested they retire simultaneously. They were both seventy-five. The whole company—all thirty employees—came to their farewell party. He got a gold watch, she got a silver one, and that was it.

Caring for her ninety-four-year-old mother was the next job she had to give up. Her mother had gradually developed dementia—whether it was Alzheimer's disease or some other form, Catherine did not know. The result was that she forgot whether she had eaten, forgot to change her clothes, and left the stove on. The final straw was when she went for a walk in her nightgown in the middle of a typical New England February night. She had outlived two of her own children, Catherine's sister and brother. Reluctantly, Catherine put her mother in a nursing home.

The weekly Sunday evening dinners for the family were not the same after her mother was institutionalized. The grandchildren no longer came regularly, and Andrea and Jennifer felt it was too much for their mother to prepare an elaborate meal, even for five. After a series of excuses for not coming—one week Jennifer was too tired, the next week her husband was away on a business trip; then Andrea was attending her twenty-fifth college reunion and the following week her husband had a cold—Catherine gave up. Not only did she abandon any effort to get the family together for dinner, but she also decided it was time to sell the house. The triple-decker had served the family well for years: it had been the ideal setup during the years of Maury's disability, when he had survived thanks to his sister-in-law above and his mother-in-law below. Now Catherine's sister was dead, her mother was in a nursing home, and she herself did not need the six large, high-ceilinged rooms that made up the middle story. The neighborhood had changed as well: instead of the lower-middle-class suburb it had been when her father had bought his home, it was now a working-class neighborhood of new immigrant families. Unhappy with her responsibilities as a landlady, rattling around in the huge apartment with no friends in the neighborhood, Catherine decided to move.

Once she moved, it was impractical to remain as president of the senior center. She lived in a different town now, separated from her origins by a mere ten miles in physical distance, but by a spiritual chasm. Her new home was a one-bedroom apartment in a senior citizens' complex. Over the course of a few months, Catherine Endicott retired four times.

Always the optimist, always a hard worker, and never one to remain idle for long, she began volunteering at the local library. It was just a three-block walk and she went only twice a week, weather permitting. Instead of cooking for her daughters, she allowed them to take her out to dinner on alternating weeks. Her hearing had deteriorated, so she preferred dinner with one table-mate to a whole gathering. Instead of keeping the books for the Martin J. Smith Dry Goods Company, she concentrated on keeping her own household in order. And in place of caring for her ailing mother, she focused on caring for herself.

Because of a failing heart, Catherine tired easily. She got short of breath when climbing stairs, and was grateful that she lived in an elevator building. She found that everything took her twice as long as previously: she was often constipated, and had to sit in the bathroom for extended periods of time. She could not walk the three blocks to the library without a rest, so she devised a strategy of stopping midway at a drugstore, ostensibly to buy a newspaper. On the way home, she paused at a convenience store, managing to find that she had run out of milk or soap. It was always a small item she needed, so as not to have to lug a heavy shopping bag home. At the relatively young age of seventy-five, Catherine Endicott had become frail.

Jack Simon

Jack Simon did not slide gradually into frailty: he went from vigor to dependence overnight. He had been working until the day he had the stroke.

"I never really retired from my business," Jack explained to me. "It was too big a part of my life. I started there when I was just a kid, really. I had wanted to be a medical professional, a podiatrist actually, but then the Depression came along and I had to help support my parents and my sisters. I was lucky to get a job. I started out in the factory, assembling boxes. I rose in the ranks, becoming a supervisor after just a couple of years. And then I moved into sales. I was a damned good salesman. I was with the same company my whole career."

"I stepped down from sales when I turned seventy, but I still went to the office a few times a week as a consultant. And then on the side I set up a new business, as a sort of career counselor to executives in their fifties who had lost their jobs. I was always upbeat, had a positive attitude, which lots of these fellas really needed. A good outlook and a well-done résumé and a lot of perseverance—that's what it takes to find a new job after you've been laid off at age fifty." He paused for a moment, and then refocused. "That's what I was doing—still putting in two days a week at the office and a couple of days on my second career, right up to my eightieth birthday. They had quite a birthday bash for me—mainly family, but some guys from the company and a few of my advisees, too. Dinner and dancing at a nice hotel. It was kind of like a wedding. Don't think I just watched—I danced plenty. A week later, I woke up in the middle of the night and had to go to the bathroom but I couldn't get up. First I thought my arm was asleep. Then I realized my whole side didn't move. I tried calling to my wife, but I couldn't talk right. My speech was all jangled up. Finally, Peggy heard me and came in. She took one look at me and she knew I'd had a stroke."[7]

Jack was in the hospital for a week and then in a rehabilitation facility for another six weeks. He made extraordinary progress. His speech was almost normal: apart from occasional difficulty finding words, he was quite fluent. He exercised as instructed and regained considerable strength in his arm and leg, but not enough to walk. Jack was determined to become independent once again, and succeeded in learning to transfer from a wheelchair to the toilet, and from his bed to a chair. After a month of intensive work, he stabilized, making no further gains.

The rehab staff was convinced that Jack would need to be in a nursing home, but his wife, Margaret, was equally convinced that he would be able to manage at home. The problem, the physical therapist tried to state as diplomatically as possible, was that Jack was six feet tall and weighed 200 pounds. Margaret was a petite five feet four inches, svelte at 105 pounds. While she was in excellent shape for her seventy-eight years—she walked two miles every day in good weather and peddled five miles on her exercise bike in bad—she clearly would not be able to lift Jack off the toilet or from a wheelchair into bed.

"But I don't have to be able to lift him," Margaret protested. "We agreed that if he could transfer himself, he could come home." Over and over, Jack demonstrated to the therapists' satisfaction that he could, in fact, transfer himself. The only transfer he still had difficulty with was into a car.

"So we won't go anywhere," Margaret said flatly. "If he went to a nursing home he wouldn't go anywhere, either. But in a nursing home, 'home' would be a place he wouldn't want to be. If he stays in the house, I'll have to get a chair car for medical appointments. Or my kids will help. I have two sons who are built just like their father."

"What if he falls? You won't be able to get him off the floor."

"He won't fall," Margaret responded, her eyes flashing and her lips set in a determined line.

The physical therapist, who worked on Jack's walking and his balance, and the occupational therapist, who helped him learn to get dressed and washed, made a visit to the Simons' home. Their task was to determine what adaptive equipment the Simons would need to enable Jack to try living at home.

The house was a tidy three-bedroom colonial. "Six steps just to get inside," the physical therapist commented as soon as she arrived. "And all the bedrooms are upstairs. Where's Jack going to sleep?"

Margaret had everything figured out. She would convert the first-floor family room, which they hadn't used since the children had grown up, into a bedroom. Fortunately, there was a half-bath on the same level. The only bathtub was upstairs, but it would take a lift to get Jack in and out of a tub anyway. He could benefit from a stall shower, which they didn't have. If the arrangements worked out, Margaret would have one built in the downstairs bathroom. The plumbing was already there, and the wall to the adjoining closet could be knocked down to create enough space. In the meantime, Jack would take sponge baths.

The physical therapist whipped out a tape measure to see if the first-floor hallways were wide enough to accommodate a wheelchair. "Barely adequate," she muttered.

The living room was far too cluttered with furniture to allow Jack to maneuver in his wheelchair. "No problem," Margaret said, recognizing that the therapist was absolutely right. "I'll get rid of that old sofa. The bookcases I can put upstairs since we won't be using our old bedroom."

"These throw rugs are a hazard—too easy to trip on, if Jack starts walking again. They're very nice, though," she added, not wishing to appear overly negative. "A commode for the new bedroom would be a good idea, so Jack won't have to go far during the night. You'll need a few grab bars for the walls here and there."

A week later, Jack came home. His three children had flown in to greet him. Mark, who was a graphic designer, had made a huge WELCOME HOME, DAD banner. Ginny had baked an enormous cake. Stuart, the youngest, had made a ramp for the front steps. All three of them had worked to move furniture around. Jack had tears in his eyes when he saw what they had done for him.

"You're such great kids—that's what makes it all worthwhile." Margaret hid her tears. That was as close as Jack had come to acknowledging that he hadn't been uniformly convinced during his hospitalizations that life was still worth living.

They celebrated all afternoon and all evening. First they ate the cake. When they worked up an appetite again, Jack had Chinese food delivered for dinner. They all laughed and joked and watched old home movies that anyone else would have found extremely tedious. That first night, the kids slept in their old bedrooms upstairs to be on hand for any problems.

There were no problems. They continued celebrating and visiting the next day. Mark went over some financial matters with his father, and Ginny went out shopping so her mother would have everything she needed for at least a week. Stuart got the car inspected—that had always been his father's job, but Jack would no longer be driving. There were countless things to attend to that Margaret had put off while Jack was at the rehab facility. With everyone working together, the mountain on Margaret's desk was whittled down to a molehill. And then it was time for the children to say good-bye. Promising to call and to visit, and exhorting their parents to let them know if they could help, they went back to their usual lives—their jobs, their spouses, their own children. Margaret and Jack were by themselves in the house.

The first night they were alone, Margaret hardly slept. For

more than two months she had not been alone with Jack. Not truly alone. There had been nurses, doctors, therapists. Then there had been the children, strong, capable, and efficient. Suddenly, Margaret was on her own. She lay in bed, the dubious expression on the visiting therapist's face looming before her. She felt out of place sleeping, or trying to sleep, in the newly fashioned downstairs bedroom. She wasn't sure she would be able to manage.

By light of day, the situation seemed far less ominous. Margaret felt much more confident. None of the tasks facing her seemed particularly daunting. One after another, friends and neighbors stopped by to see Jack, usually bringing food and offers to help. The following day, three of his "students" visited—executives whose careers he had helped redirect. They brought an inspired and touching gift: realizing that Jack would have trouble using his computer in view of the weakness in his right hand, they had bought him speech-recognition software. After a brief training session, he would be able to dictate to his computer, barely using his hands. Their faith in Jack's continued ability to work moved him to tears for the second time since his return home.

After a week, the calls and visits had slowed down. Margaret and Jack were truly on their own. "I have to do some food shopping," Margaret noted worriedly one morning, when she realized they were out of orange juice.

"Well, go ahead."

"But I—I don't want to leave you alone."

"Why not? I'll be fine."

"What if something happens?"

"If what happens?"

"If you need help. If you fall."

"If I fall, you wouldn't be able to pick me up in any case."

"I could phone for help, though."

"Margaret, have I fallen this past week?"

"No."

"Have I gotten stuck in the bathroom?"

"No."

"Okay. So relax. I'm just going to sit in this chair while you're out, watching the news. Now go."

Margaret went, but she was inordinately anxious. She rushed back in record time. She resolved to go out only to do errands, never for pleasure. She arranged for Jack to be connected to Life Line: he would wear a device around his neck that would enable him to summon assistance by pressing a button if he got into difficulty while she was away. Jack thought the entire arrangement excessive, but it afforded Margaret a little peace of mind.

Not much peace of mind. Not enough to allow her to go to a movie with friends or to accept an invitation for a day on the beach. When her daughter offered to take her to her summer cottage on Cape Cod for a weekend, Margaret was appalled. She could not conceive of leaving Jack alone at night and certainly not for a whole weekend. He was no longer the capable, self-reliant man she had married. He looked the same as he had six months earlier, he sounded the same, but he had been transformed. If there was a slight perturbation in his health or a malfunction in the external systems on which he relied to get by, he would be a mess. His enlarged prostate, for instance, had been a minor annoyance for several years. There were days when he had to go to the bathroom frequently and urgently. With his new mobility problems, he could not go anywhere quickly. As a result, he had several distressing bladder "accidents." In a similar vein, Jack found that the marked decrease in his activity level led to severe constipation. Before he understood what had happened and how to prevent it, matters got so bad that a nurse had to come to his home to give him an enema. He went on a daily prune regime with good results, but had to remember that he was predisposed to recurrences. Whenever he took Tylenol with codeine for headaches, he was at risk of getting bound up all over again. He simply had to be more vigilant about his plumbing than ever before.

Jack and Margaret were managing at home, but they both understood just what frailty was all about.

Leyla Keribar

Valerie never imagined her mother would move in with her permanently. Her friends laugh and say it was inevitable. As soon as the decision was made that Leyla and Imre Keribar would leave their native Turkey and move to the United States, it was natural to conclude that they would stay with their daughter. "Of course, I knew they would stay in the beginning," Valerie explained, "but I didn't think they would remain indefinitely. I guess somehow I expected that even though they were in their sixties and Dad was a sick man and mother had never held a paying job, they would make it on their own."

When Imre died a few years after the move, it went without saying that his widow would remain in Valerie's house. Why would she move out once she was alone if she hadn't when she had a spouse? Valerie and her husband, George, had gone so far as to move to a new, larger house two years before Imre's death so that each generation could have its privacy. The new house—as Leyla would always refer to it—had a small garden apartment on the lower level. The suite included a bedroom, a sitting room, and a bath, and opened onto a stone patio set in a secluded, tastefully designed garden. Valerie, who was an interior decorator, furnished the apartment and decorated it to suit her parents' needs.

Leyla never appreciated the new arrangement. In the first manifestation of what would prove to be her growing cantankerousness, she harangued her daughter and son-in-law for moving. She felt she had been "exiled" to the garden apartment. Whereas previously she had been completely integrated into the family, sharing the only living room, sleeping in a bedroom on the second floor among all the other bedrooms, now she had her own space. She still ate most of her meals with Valerie and George, but she felt abandoned. She called her apartment the "maid's quarters" and professed incomprehension at Valerie's decision to move just when her sons were getting ready to go off to college. Other women would have enjoyed the combination of privacy and togetherness that the garden apartment offered. Leyla complained. In fact, she protested the very concept of being alone.

The fear of being alone reached new heights when Valerie and George decided to go on a trip abroad for a month. Their children had never been to Turkey, where their mother had grown up and their grandparents had lived most of their lives. The children were fifteen and seventeen, perched on the brink of adulthood. They were old enough to appreciate learning about their heritage. They also happened to be at a point in their development where they found their parents' company quite tolerable. Unlike some of their friends, they were willing to be seen in public with their parents. They had no plans of their own that summer, so the four Lewises took off for Turkey.

Valerie left a dozen precooked dinners in the freezer for her mother. She arranged for groceries to be delivered every week while she was away and asked their neighbor to check up on Leyla. When she returned home, Valerie knew at once that something was wrong. The house was subtly changed. Not dirty, certainly not smelly, not even disorderly. Things were ever so slightly out of place: a dishtowel instead of a face cloth in the bathroom, the flowery cushions on the living room sofa swapped for the striped cushions in the den. A stick of margarine and a half dozen eggs were stashed away in the freezer.

Had Leyla lost her bearings? Was she losing touch with reality? Valerie grilled her neighbor. No, nothing was unequivocally wrong, but nothing was entirely right either. Leyla had been very quiet whenever he had come over. She had responded politely to his questions, usually in monosyllables. She had not once invited him in for coffee or tea. On one occasion, when he had stopped by after doing some errands, he had complained about the stultifying humidity, the hot, motionless air, and the pollen count.

"It's brutal out there," he had told Leyla. "Do you have air-conditioning?"

"A fan," she had answered cursorily.

"We got central air last year. It's a blessing in weather like this. Are you all right here?"

"Fine."

"Do you think, do you have—could I have a glass of ice water?" her neighbor finally blurted out.

"Of course." Leyla gestured toward the kitchen but offered no assistance as he searched through the cabinets for a tumbler. She did not follow him into the kitchen, but hovered at the doorway, watching him with her large brown eyes. If he noticed the eggs in the freezer when he took out the ice cubes, he didn't say anything. He drank his water and left, glad to retreat into the heat. Unbearable weather was normal in New England in August. Something about Leyla was not.

"I came back a couple of days later, this time in the morning. She was up and dressed and said she'd had breakfast. Nothing seemed out of the ordinary. I figured she just didn't want me there."

Valerie thanked him for his attentiveness and reassured him

that her mother was behaving in the same remote manner with her. "I'm going to take her to the doctor's for a checkup," Valerie told him.

The doctor performed a brief examination, ordered a few tests, and pronounced his verdict. "It's just the Parkinson's: she moves slowly, and she doesn't have much facial expression. That's classic for Parkinson's. It's easy to mistake for some other problem," he said smugly.[8] Patients and their families were forever reporting on little quirks—observations they took to be highly significant. They looked to the physician to figure out the meaning of every little twinge or ache. Usually the symptom was not nearly as momentous as the patient thought: that chronic cough was due to postnasal drip, not lung cancer; that heartburn indicated a mild case of reflux, not an ulcer. Leyla Keribar's case, he was confident, was another instance of a family mistaking a routine manifestation of a common condition for a much more ominous disease.

One day after that visit to the doctor, Valerie returned home from work to an unnaturally silent house. Her mother was a quiet person, but she often listened to music. The fan was usually on. Within moments of her unlocking the door, Leyla, who had extremely acute hearing, would wend her way from the garden apartment to greet her daughter. On that day, Valerie recalled, she strained to hear the slight shuffle of her mother's sandals, but heard nothing.

"Mom?"

No response.

"Mother? I'm home!"

A stillness, an eerie silence.

Valerie hurried to her mother's sitting room. She marveled for an instant at what a lovely job she had done with the interior decorating. Glass sliders opened to the deck. The walls were painted blue. The blue of the room blended in with the blue of the sky to give the impression of vastness, of being outside. A rubber tree in the corner and a table full of plants contributed to the blurring between indoors and out. Finding the living room unoccupied, Valerie continued into the bedroom.

At first glance, her mother appeared to be asleep. She was lying on the bed, motionless. "Mother?" she called out again.

Still no response. Valerie went over to the bed and nudged her mother gently. She was breathing quietly, slowly. She did not awaken. Then Valerie noticed the pill boxes on her night table. One was her Sinemet, the Parkinson's medication. One was Tylenol with codeine, left over from when Imre used painkillers. The last was a container of antianxiety medication. They were all empty.

"Mother!" Valerie called out one more time, shaking her vigorously. Nothing. The seriousness of the situation must have hit Valerie then, though she could not remember dialing 911 for an ambulance, or what she did while she waited for the medics. She must have called her husband, because he joined her at the hospital within an hour. She must have gathered the pill boxes into her handbag, because she had them to show the doctors in the emergency room.

The next twenty-four hours were touch and go. The doctors pumped out Leyla's stomach. They administered a thick slurry of charcoal through a nasogastric tube to bind whatever pills were no longer in the stomach but had not yet passed into her bloodstream. They put a tube into her lungs, attached to a mechanical ventilator, to breathe for her since her own breaths were shallow and inadequate. Then they waited for her kidneys and liver to perform their customary detoxification functions. Her organs obliged, machines supporting her in the interim.

By the next morning, Leyla was waking up. She began struggling against the ventilator that was programmed to pump air into her lungs twelve times every minute. The ventilator was disconnected and Leyla breathed on her own.

The following day she was alert enough to talk to a psychiatrist. No, she hadn't really meant to kill herself. She had merely wanted to have a long sleep. What gave her pleasure in life? Nothing. How did she see herself? As a useless old woman. Would anyone be sad if she died? Her daughter would be sad, but then she would feel relieved to be rid of the old hag.[9]

Valerie was shocked and hurt. She had never resented her mother. She had schemed to bring her to the United States from Turkey, and had invited her to live with her own family. She had moved to a new home so that her mother could have more privacy. Nothing had been enough. Valerie and Leyla both began psychotherapy. Leyla also took antidepressant medication for a few months, but she couldn't tolerate the side effects. Those were the pre-Prozac days, Valerie mused, thinking back.

For the next year, Leyla's depression remained reasonably well controlled. But very gradually, her Parkinson's got worse. She became shaky at unpredictable moments. She did not trust herself to handle hot pots or to put dishes in the oven. Even drinking a cup of hot coffee triggered tremendous anxiety. Besides, Leyla was uncomfortable in her daughter's ultramodern kitchen. She had never learned to use the microwave oven, and she was frightened of the Cuisinart. Valerie tried to explain to her mother that the electric can opener made life easier for someone like her, with arthritis, but Leyla found it intimidating. Leyla's main joy in life apart from her family and her piano playing had been traveling downtown, meeting friends for tea, and serving as a lunch monitor at the local elementary school. Her mobility was too precarious for her to take public transportation, and she did not drive. The net result was that she stayed home all day, a frail old lady who ventured forth only when her daughter and son-in-law took her out with them.

Ben Frank, Catherine Endicott, Jack Simon, and Leyla Keribar followed markedly different roads to frailty. Ben Frank descended along a gently sloping path, barely aware that he was losing altitude. Catherine Endicott proceeded along a stepwise descent, suffering discrete, significant reverses with each cardiac event, then cruising along on a plateau for a while, only to have another acute episode that caused her to move down another step. Jack Simon fell off a precipice and found himself in the land of frailty, though he managed to pull himself up a few notches from the gorge in which he landed. Leyla Keribar found herself proceeding along a moderately steep path, and then took a detour down another road with a sharper incline when depression supervened.

Because their journeys were so different, their awareness of what was happening to them varied. Ben Frank was caught up in the minutiae of his medications and his new symptoms and was not in a position to step back and observe that his sense of well-being, his day-to-day functioning, and his overall health had changed between his eighty-first and eighty-second birthdays. His physicians shared his perspective, focusing on each acute problem as it arose and never assessing the toll of those events on the whole person. Catherine Endicott adapted so well to each small decrement in her cardiac status that the full magnitude of her frailty was not evident for some time. Jack Simon was well aware that he had entered a new phase of his life, but he was so busy trying to overcome his deficits, trying to repair all that he had lost, which proved impossible, that it was a while before he adjusted to his new condition. Leyla Keribar sensed that she was losing her independence and became anxious out of proportion to her physical disability.

Having achieved the status of frailty, all four had to make major adjustments in their approach to living. They needed to come to grips with the fact that while they could not regain their previous condition, they could often significantly improve their lot by modifying one component of their frailty. Poor vision, or chest pain, or hearing loss, were, if anything, more important to attend to than if they had been vigorous, because of the interrelatedness of the factors conspiring to produce frailty. They needed to examine their living situation and make major changes—in some cases moving out, and in some cases finding a caregiver to move in—since their environment could either hamper or facilitate their functioning. When they developed further medical problems—and all four were destined to have additional serious bodily malfunctions necessitating extensive interactions with the medical profession—they had to struggle with how much technology was appropriate for them. Modern medicine, they would learn, can sometimes, though not always, cure what were once lethal ailments, but the price is often a deeper descent into frailty. While some people opt for attempts at life-prolongation, regardless of the consequences for their level of functioning or their likelihood of success, others are reluctant to plunge further into frailty.

Ben Frank, Catherine Endicott, Jack Simon, and Leyla Keribar each faced physical challenges, but they also faced spiritual challenges. They struggled to find meaning in their lives despite their losses, their dependence on others, and their inability to derive sustenance from their customary endeavors. They found their own ways, through family, through volunteering, through friendship. When they did not find their way, they tended to lapse into despair.

Coming to terms with frailty is a family enterprise, not merely an individual challenge. The children, and in some cases the spouse, of the affected person, must learn a new role. Once the beneficiaries of parental caregiving, offspring must learn to help take care of their sometimes reluctant parents. Often, just when they find themselves liberated from parenting responsibilities, they are asked to take on similar responsibilities for their own parents. The adult children are called upon to handle finances, to orchestrate medical care, to participate in decisions about limiting care. One of the first dilemmas that family members face as their relatives journey through frailty is whether to fix various bodily parts as they begin to break down.

CHAPTER 2

Fixing the Fixable Part

The encouraging news about frailty is that even though it typically cannot be cured, modest improvements in any of its component parts can have a dramatic effect on the whole person. An individual with four chronic illnesses often derives more mileage from amelioration of a single symptom than does her counterpart who has only one problem. The reason for this seeming paradox is that the four conditions interact with each other in such a way that worsening of one may trigger deterioration in all the others. Put differently, the frail person has difficulty maintaining homeostasis, or internal-organ equilibrium. Frailty has been characterized as homeostenosis, or a loss of the normal adaptability of the organism. A seemingly minor perturbation of the system can have major consequences. Repairing that small problem produces correspondingly potent results.

The implication of these observations is that certain kinds of problems in the frail person are critical to address—promptly. Failing to fix a fixable problem can lead to a downward spiral that may be difficult or impossible to reverse. Conversely, a timely intervention can make an enormous difference in the ability to function, to cope, and to enjoy life.

Ben Frank

Susan came over for dinner. We chatted about work, about vacations, about her upcoming art exhibit. Before we got to dessert, the conversation moved to family. We talked about Susan's brother, who had remained single until age forty and then surprised her by getting married and having a child. We talked about my boys, comparing the world in which they were growing up (very focused on the here and now) to the world as it was when we were children (future-oriented). And then, inevitably, Susan mentioned her father.

"I went to New York to visit him last weekend. I couldn't talk to him on the phone anymore—he just can't hear me. Face-to-face is okay, as long as the radio is off. Though actually it's a disaster if there are several people in the room—Dad doesn't know where to turn. Unless he's looking right at you and you're looking at him, he just can't understand."

"He probably reads lips a lot more than he realizes," I commented.

"I guess so. My brother and his wife and my niece came to visit one afternoon, and it was pathetic. Eventually he just tuned out, retreated into his shell. He just sat there. He actually didn't look unhappy—but, then, he's such a stoic. He doesn't expect he could actually be together with his family and talk to them."

We discussed getting a special telephone for him on which

the volume can be adjusted. I also broached the subject of a hearing aid.

"He won't wear one. He says they're no good. My mother had hearing aids in both ears and she often didn't hear what we said. But with her, the problem was that she didn't pay attention. Dad is different. He listens—he just can't hear."

"Do you think he's self-conscious?" I asked. Many people are embarrassed about wearing hearing aids, even though the contemporary versions, both those in the ear and those behind the ear, are quite inconspicuous.

"My father was never a vain man," Susan said defensively.

"Still," I pressed, "lots of people feel awkward appearing in public with a cane, let alone a walker. They are uncomfortable admitting they have any kind of handicap."

"You would think he would be more self-conscious about the fact that he has to ask you to repeat yourself or that he says things that don't make any sense because he is answering a question you didn't ask."

"He probably doesn't know that he wasn't answering the right question. And people have a tremendous capacity for rationalization—he probably thinks there's an epidemic of quiet speech."

Susan laughed, and admitted that perhaps her father was denying he had a problem. She agreed to begin by working on getting a new telephone for him and then tackling the question of a hearing test.

Unfortunately, Ben Frank was right that hearing aids are far from perfect. They do not restore hearing with anything approaching the fidelity with which glasses restore vision. Hearing aids distort, but despite their inadequacies, they can make a tremendous difference in social functioning.

Ben was a hard sell. He did accept the amplified telephone. I suspected his acquiescence indicated both that he recognized he had a problem and that he was more comfortable with an adaptive device that was hidden from view than with one that he wore on his head. The special phone worked well, but did not lead him to conclude that a hearing aid would likewise be useful. Instead, he became increasingly reclusive. The few social activities he had come to enjoy since his wife's death—visiting the local men's club and going to the movies—he abandoned. He had excuses for everything that had nothing to do with his hearing: the only men he liked at the club had either died or moved to Florida; Hollywood made movies about gay men and unattached professional women, neither of whom he could relate to.

Susan was convinced that her father was becoming depressed. The signs were subtle. His bedtime, usually ten o'clock, began creeping back, first to nine, then to eight. Susan, who had a busy life involving choral groups and art classes, rarely got home before nine, so she found she could never call her father in the evenings. Even though he claimed he didn't mind being awakened, his thinking was so muddled after he first woke up that Susan found it frustrating to talk to him. Ben also began losing weight because he had lost interest in eating. His daughter discovered just how much weight he had lost when his birthday rolled around. She gave him her usual gift, a pair of chinos carefully selected from the L.L. Bean catalog. They were the same size she had ordered each of the previous three years, but they were hopelessly wide. He claimed he was contented with his lot, but his appetite was poor, he slept all the time, and during his few waking hours he sat at home doing nothing. He watched his homemaker do household chores. He did his own laundry and paid the bills. His only pleasure in life, aside from visits from his children, was reading *The New York Times,* which he did faithfully and in its entirety.

Susan worried that persuading her father to speak to his

physician about taking an antidepressant would be just as formidable an undertaking as persuading him to accept a special telephone had been. She reluctantly took the distasteful step of calling the doctor directly, imploring him not to breathe a word of their conversation to her dad, and then outlining the reasons for her concern. He was dubious at first: he thought all old people go to bed at eight (they don't); he blamed the poor appetite on the low-salt, low-fat diet he had prescribed (Ben Frank had never paid the slightest attention to the doctor's dietary recommendations); and he thought that the restricted social life was a part of the "disengagement" that is normal in the elderly (a largely discredited myth).[1] When Ben stepped on the scale at his next appointment and weighed ten pounds less than he had three months earlier, Dr. Andrews recalled his conversation with Susan. After he could find no anemia or bloody stools or hormonal imbalance to explain the weight loss, he agreed to put Ben on an antidepressant.

Dr. Andrews was a conservative physician who believed that tried-and-true medications were preferable to newfangled drugs. This attitude is usually auspicious in caring for elderly patients, though occasionally it is an excuse for failing to learn about the newest developments in medicine. In the arena of psychiatric medications, Dr. Andrews was particularly cautious. He prescribed nortriptyline for Ben Frank, a tricyclic antidepressant that had been on the market for decades. It was a wise choice, for a tricyclic, since it was relatively nonsedating and had less of a tendency to cause confusion than did some of its cousins. But compared to serotonin reuptake inhibitors, drugs like Prozac and Zoloft, it was more likely to cause a dry mouth, constipation, and difficulty urinating.

After five days on the new medication, Ben began to have trouble going to the bathroom. First it was his bowels—uncom-

fortable and distressing but rapidly responsive to over-the-count-
er milk of magnesia. Then it was his bladder, which did not
respond to any of his home remedies. He tried drinking a lot of
fluid, which just made matters worse because he developed a mas-
sively distended bladder and still could not void. Eventually he
was in so much pain he called 911 and was transported by ambulance to the local hospital emergency room. A catheter was
threaded through his penis and into his bladder, providing instant
relief. The catheter was then removed and he was promptly sent
home, with the none-too-reassuring warning that if he didn't successfully pass urine in eight hours, he should come back for
another catheterization. His problem was attributed to an
enlarged prostate that was believed to be obstructing the outflow
of urine from the bladder. Ben was given a referral to a urologist
and told he would in all likelihood need prostate surgery.[2]

Ben Frank *did* have benign prostatic hyperplasia (an enlarged
but noncancerous prostate gland), and his prostate *was* contributing to his difficulty passing urine. The missing piece in the explanation, however, was that until he began taking nortriptyline, his
bladder had been working just fine. The nortriptyline had not
done anything to his prostate, nor had his prostate suddenly
enlarged. The medication worked on the bladder wall, diminish-
ing the strength of its contractions. This modest effect, in combination with the mild chronic narrowing from his enlarged
prostate, was just enough to push Ben into full-blown urinary
retention.

The next twenty-four hours were decidedly unpleasant. Ben
managed to stay out of the emergency room, but barely. He discovered that if he massaged his lower abdomen, he could literally
push out the urine. He was so distraught that he forgot to take
his medications. He went to the urology clinic of the hospital at
which he had been catheterized, where he had to wait two hours

to be seen. At the end of the two hours, during which he fre-
quented the men's room half a dozen times, always worried that
he would be called while he was busy pressing, coaxing, and ultimately partially emptying his bladder, he was examined by a urology resident, fresh out of a general surgery residency. From the
resident's perspective, the only question was whether to put in a
catheter and leave it in until the date of surgery. Ben was adamant
that he wasn't going to go home with a tube dangling from his
penis, and the resident could not justify admitting him to the
hospital until the operation. Rather doubtful of his new patient's
wisdom, he sent him home with "semielective" surgery scheduled
for one week later.

Ben Frank hastily concluded that the antidepressant medication was not working. He stopped the nortriptyline for the wrong
reason: perversely, insufficient time had elapsed to declare the
medication a failure in treating his depression, but ample time
had passed for the pills to work their mischief on his bladder. To
Ben's surprise and the urology resident's astonishment, each day
it was easier to start a stream. One day before he was supposed to
go in for a transurethral prostatectomy, Ben found he could
empty his bladder completely and without difficulty. He canceled
the surgery and announced to his daughter that he had lost whatever little faith he had had in the medical profession.

Susan called me from New York. She had gone there for the
weekend to celebrate her father's eighty-third birthday and was at
her wits' end. The party had been low key, but it had been a party:
ten people crammed into her father's two-bedroom apartment for
coffee and cake. Ben had not understood a word anyone had said.
He smiled benevolently at his family and seemed to enjoy his
cake. He had always been a fairly passive person, at least by comparison with his domineering wife. To see him sitting amid his
relatives, physically present but spiritually absent, Susan found

intolerable. She excused herself before the party was over and took the train into Manhattan to visit the Museum of Modern Art. The dissonant, harsh images of the paintings jibed with her angry, helpless mood. By the time she got back to her father's apartment in the Bronx, he had gone to bed.

"It's all so unnecessary!"

"Maybe he was still pleased that everyone came," I suggested.

"Oh, he was pleased all right. But he could actually have used his brain instead of just sitting there if he'd been able to hear. My cousin Adam was there—he's a journalist and he just came back from Thailand. He has all sorts of fascinating stories to tell. Adam told him the government denied there had been a single case of AIDS in Thailand, even though it's rampant among Thai prostitutes, who are now infecting foreign tourists. My dad nodded and said he was glad America was giving *aid* to Thailand. He came across as such an idiot!"

"I'm sure everyone realized he couldn't hear."

"I'm not so sure. My cousins haven't visited in a while. Actually, I think they thought he was senile—demented."

We talked about dementia for a while—I was fleetingly concerned that he might in fact have cognitive difficulties. Frequently family members mistake a failing mind for hearing loss. Susan assured me that, one-on-one, her father's thinking was entirely normal.

"Perhaps it's time for you and your brother to sit down with your father and read him the riot act. I know he doesn't have a lot of faith in doctors right now, but at this point what he needs is an audiologist to do a hearing test, not a physician."

As we spoke, I thought of a patient of mine who had benefited tremendously from an amplifier, or pocket talker. The device, available at consumer electronics stores, involves earphones attached to a handheld unit that has a built-in microphone. The gadget can be passed from one speaker to another, allowing the wearer to hear not only one-on-one, but also in a group setting. My patient also had hearing aids, but her hearing was so profoundly impaired that she did better with the pocket talker, whereby the person speaking did so directly into the microphone. I told Susan about the gadget. She decided instantly that she would buy one and bring it with her on her next trip to New York.

My next phone call from Susan was remarkably upbeat. She had bought the pocket talker. Her father had used it, though reluctantly, and only with immediate family, which meant Susan and her brother. But the result had been so astonishing that he actually agreed to an audiologic evaluation. He allowed himself to be fitted for a hearing aid—an inconspicuous in-the-ear device. The struggle was not over: he often forgot to put in the hearing aids, particularly when he needed them most, when he was with groups of people. There was no question that he was embarrassed to be seen with them. He even started wearing a hat and pulling the flaps down to keep his ears out of view. He had difficulty learning to change the batteries, and sometimes he rammed the right hearing aid into the left ear and then complained bitterly that the things didn't work properly and gave him an earache. At the beginning, he did not adjust the volume appropriately, and suffered from the whines and screeches characteristic of excessive feedback. But gradually Ben got used to the hearing aids. He began to wear them regularly. He learned how to set the volume correctly and change the batteries. Very slowly, he started to go out more, to do more. Susan knew she had won the battle when she took her father to a movie and he insisted on going home and returning for a later show because he had left his hearing aids at home.

. . .

Once Ben Frank began venturing out of his apartment again, he did something he hadn't done in forty years, Susan told me. It was nothing extravagant, like buying himself a cashmere coat. It was nothing romantic, like taking a woman on a harbor cruise. Nonetheless, for Ben it was quite extraordinary. He made a friend.

Not that Ben hadn't had friends during his married life. He had had quite a few friends—family friends, relatives, neighborhood friends. But his wife had always taken the initiative. When they went on vacation, she struck up a conversation with the couple seated next to them in the dining room. When they joined the tenants' group in their apartment building, his wife did all the talking. She joined a bridge club, she made conversation in the elevator. When friends came over for dinner, or they went to the movies together, Ben joined in the conversation. But he always felt their visitors were his wife's friends. They had all come to her funeral and then dropped out of his life.

It happened on a mild autumn afternoon, when Ben went for a brief walk. He tired easily—whether it was an ache in his calves or shortness of breath he couldn't say, but after a block or two he felt he needed to rest. He stopped at a bench, conveniently situated along the main thoroughfare, overlooking a patch of grass about four feet by five feet, on which was planted a small sign implausibly proclaiming it as SERGEANT MORIARTY PARK. Another man was already sitting on the bench, shabbily dressed in a worn leather jacket, faded corduroy pants, and old sneakers. Like Ben, he was wearing a tweed cap.

The length of the bench separated the two men, as was customary between strangers on a New York City bench. Ben thought the other man was sleeping and was surprised when he started to speak, barely opening his eyes.

"Nice day, isn't it?" the other man said.

"Very nice," Ben agreed.

"After all that rain, it's good to see the sun," the man commented.

"Warm, too," Ben added.

"For autumn, it sure is," the other man said.

That exhausted their store of sociability. After a few minutes, Ben stood up, ready to head back home. This time, he was certain his benchmate had dozed off. He was breathing slowly and evenly. His mouth was slightly open.

"Have a good day," the man called after Ben. Ben doffed his hat in return.

When they met again on the same bench the following day, their conversation was devoted to exploring this remarkable coincidence.

"You again! Do you come here every day?" the man asked.

"Not when it's raining."

"Of course not. I don't either. But on a sunny day like this . . ."

"It's quite something we should have come out at just the same time," Ben remarked. "Almost as though we were waiting for the same bus."

"Are you waiting for the bus?"

"No, no. I'm just resting. I meant—we're like two guys who meet every day because they always take the same commuter train."

"Except that we're not waiting for a train."

"Except that we're not waiting for a train," Ben repeated. "Or a bus," he added, lest his words be interpreted literally.

"I'm not waiting for anything," the stranger commented. "Just getting a little fresh air before the frost sets in. It's going to be a long winter."

Ben agreed. He hadn't given any thought before this to how many months he would be cooped up during the winter, when

the ground was too icy or the weather too stormy to venture outside.

"I guess I won't see you anymore when it gets very cold," Ben
observed.

"I suppose not. Though you might not see me anymore even
if it stays mild like this. It's just chance we met again today."

"That's true," Ben agreed. "Though maybe we're on the same
schedule. Get up at the same time. Eat breakfast at the same time.
Go to the store. You know, have a similar routine."

"You're quite a talker." The man turned and looked at Ben. It
had been a long time since anyone described Ben as loquacious.
Ben smiled and got up to go.

For the next week, they did not see each other. Then, while
paying for a box of cereal and a can of beans at the neighborhood
convenience store, Ben heard a familiar voice with a hint of a
Southern accent call out to him, "Hey, if it isn't my bench friend!"
He was buying a pack of cigarettes.

"My wife smoked," Ben told him. "All the smoking got to her
lungs. I think it killed her, though the doctors never said for
sure." That was as close as Ben could come to admonishing the
other man for smoking.

"What else have I got now besides smoking? The wife's gone.
I never see the kids. Who's going to miss me if I go up in
smoke?"

Ben couldn't say that *he* would—he was too shy and their
friendship was too new, too unformed. Wordlessly, the two men
walked over to the bench in Sergeant Moriarty Park and sat down
with their purchases.

"I wonder who Sergeant Moriarty was," Ben began.

"Couldn't have been very important if all he got was a four-
by-five strip of grass. Cemetery plot's probably bigger."

"Moriarty was the name of the master criminal in Sherlock

Holmes," Ben said. "I always associate that name with evil. I used to read Sherlock Holmes aloud to my children when they were little. I have a son and a daughter," he explained.

Suddenly the man turned to Ben. "My name's Will. William R. Merlin."

"I'm Ben. Benjamin Frank. Pleased to make your acquaintance."

William Merlin was seventy-eight and lived alone. He had worked as a clerk all his life—in a succession of small stores. He had moved to the neighborhood twenty years ago, participating in its transformation from a largely Jewish to a primarily black community. Ben and Will were both throwbacks to other times—now the area was predominantly Hispanic, with most of the Jews and blacks gone.

Ben and Will never visited each other's apartments. They did move from the bench to the local senior center when the weather got colder. They drank coffee together—Ben liked his black, and Will took milk and three sugars. They watched football games on the large-screen TV. Ben had never cared much for football, but Will provided a running commentary for him. They never made formal plans, but tacitly agreed to meet at the senior center when a game was on.

One Sunday, Will wasn't at the center at the usual time. He didn't show up at either of the next two football games. Ben checked out the bench, since it was unseasonably mild, but it was vacant. Finally, Ben asked the director of the senior center, a serious young man who had recently graduated from social work school, if he knew what had happened to Will. The man made some inquiries, and reported back to Ben that William Merlin had been hospitalized and was in fair condition.

Ben forgot to call ahead to inquire when visiting hours were. He took a cab to the hospital, and made his way to the four-bed room, where he found William Merlin, an intravenous in one arm and an oxygen mask on his face.

"Hey there, Ben. Nice of you to come."

"I—I was worried about you. Finally, they told me at the center where to find you."

"I'm in tough shape," Will told him. "Cancer. Lung cancer. That's why I figured the cigarettes couldn't hurt me anymore. I knew I had lung cancer."

Ben was taken aback. "I'm sorry."

"Don't be sorry," Will told him. "The only thing I worry about is not being able to breathe. Don't want to suffocate to death. That's how come I came in the other day. I couldn't breathe. Evidently I have bronchitis on top of the lung cancer. One lung's already shot, so if I get bronchitis, I'm in trouble. So they give me oxygen and medicine for a few days and then they'll send me home again."

Ben didn't know what to say. He wrote his phone number and address on a piece of paper and gave the sheet to Will.

The two men saw each other only a few more times before Will died.[3] They talked about their lives—their many disappointments, their few triumphs. Ben asked his friend what kept him going, how he endured his illness.

"The Lord Jesus keeps me going," Will said simply. He talked about his church, about the minister who came to see him at home, and about the ladies from the church who brought him hot meals when he was sick. "So, I'm not scared. When the end comes, the Lord Jesus will take me to a better place than this." He gestured out the window to the rundown stores across from the senior center. "What about you, Ben? What keeps you going?"

"My family, mainly. I guess I don't think about it much."

A week later, Ben saw his friend's name in the obituary column. He'd started reading the obituaries when his wife died, to keep tabs on his former friends. Two weeks later he got a package in the mail, with a note from the minister of Will's church: "Will asked me to send this to you. He said he knew you weren't Christian and didn't mean to hurt your feelings. But he thought you might find the stories uplifting, and the book was of no use to him anymore. God bless you." Enclosed was Will's copy of the New Testament.

As with many older people who suffer from hearing loss, Ben Frank suffered from social isolation and depression as a result of his impairment. About a quarter of adults over sixty-five have sufficient hearing loss to affect their quality of life, and the proportion rises to 36 percent in those over seventy-five.[4] Presbycusis, the technical name for the slow, progressive, symmetric hearing loss associated with old age, like so many geriatric conditions, appears to be multifactorial. It seems to result from the cumulative effect of noise and assorted substances that damage hearing, including certain medications, on top of a genetic predisposition. A single screening test done in the primary-care physician's office can help detect problems, since many individuals, like Ben Frank, do not recognize they have difficulty until it has produced major complications. Screening is best done with a brief questionnaire in conjunction with the use of an audioscope, a handheld instrument that tests hearing at a few different frequencies and decibel levels.[5] If the screening test is positive, the patient should be referred for audiologic evaluation. This is conducted by a professional audiologist, who will do a pure tone audiogram to look for the degree and type of hearing loss, and speech audiometry to assess the patient's ability to discriminate among different sounds. People who show improvement in their ability to understand speech when sound is amplified are appropriate candidates for a hearing aid.

The cost of hearing aids varies tremendously, from about three hundred dollars for a behind-the-ear model to twenty-five hundred dollars or more for a programmable in-the-ear variety. The more sophisticated models have the capacity to suppress background noise. Hearing aids are particularly useful for private conversation and small group situations. In a large room or amphitheater, other assistive listening devices can be very successful. A system in which a microphone is attached to an amplified transmitter that is placed close to the source of the sound can dramatically improve the signal-to-noise ratio and facilitate hearing lectures.

While hearing aids are far from perfect, controlled studies have confirmed the kinds of benefits seen in Ben Frank. In one clinical trial, hearing-impaired patients reported social and emotional handicaps as well as depression when they enrolled. Among those who were fitted for a hearing aid, the majority reported both social improvement and better communication, compared to those on the waiting list for a hearing aid.[6]

Catherine Endicott

Catherine Endicott's daughters were hopeful that someday their mother would change her mind about open heart surgery. "Maybe you wouldn't be so tired all the time, Mom, if you had your heart fixed," Andrea suggested.

"They can't 'fix' my heart," Catherine retorted. "The doctors said very clearly they couldn't do anything about all the dead heart tissue. Only a transplant can do that. I get tired because of the heart attack—the pump is weak. All they offered me was a bypass to give me clean, new arteries, new pipes, so I wouldn't get chest pain. But I don't get chest pain."

"I guess the medicines are working," Andrea conceded, a bit doubtful.

They were working, and they continued working for another year. Then, quite suddenly, Catherine Endicott began to have angina again. The first episode was on the way to the library. She got there, but she was pale and clearly in distress.

"Catherine, what is it?" the circulation librarian asked her, alarmed, as soon as she sat down behind the library desk.

"I don't feel too well." Catherine was panting.

"Can I get you something?"

"Get me—a glass of water."

The librarian gave Catherine water and hovered over her anxiously. "Should I call an ambulance?"

"No, I'll be fine," Catherine assured her colleague. She knew well how uncomfortable most healthy people were with disease or disability. She was very experienced, not only at caring for the sick but also at reassuring the well. *It was harder when you were the sick person,* she mused to herself. *Instead of attending to your own needs, listening to your own body, you had to worry about other people's mental state in the face of your pain.* "It's passing," Catherine said. "I'll be fine in another minute."

"Maybe you should go home," the librarian urged. Every so often one of the elderly patrons of the library passed out or took ill and she had to call an ambulance. The emergency medical technicians disturbed the tranquil atmosphere of the small branch library. Even when they did not turn their sirens on, they usually arrived with flashing lights. Protocol required that they take the patient out on a stretcher. The librarian would have preferred a more discrete exit. She was concerned about Catherine, but she also wanted to avoid the drama of a visit from the paramedics.

Privately, Catherine agreed that she probably should go home, but she wasn't sure how to get there. The prospect of walking those three blocks was alarming, since it was probably the walk that had triggered the pain. She thought of calling her daughters, but she did not want to be a burden to them. Both Andrea and Jennifer were working, and would need at least an hour to finish whatever they were doing and drive over. Catherine was also apprehensive about being at home by herself. For the first time, she felt scared and very much alone.

"I think I'll just stay here and do some quiet work. How about if I do some paperwork?" she volunteered. There was no way she was going to shelve books in her current condition.

For an hour, Catherine sent out overdue notices and cards announcing the availability of books that had been reserved. Then she called for a taxi and rode the three long blocks to her apartment.

Every day for the next week, Catherine Endicott developed chest pain. Sometimes she got it twice in one day. She husbanded her strength, she avoided any exertion, and still she got pain. Making her bed caused pain. Bending over to tie her shoes produced pain. She left her bed unmade and shuffled around in slippers, exchanging them for a well-worn pair of pumps if she went out. She walked no farther than the mailbox at the street corner, a distance of about a hundred feet, on level ground, which she found she could traverse without difficulty.

Perhaps the worst part was not knowing when the pain would hit. The predictable pain she could deal with, by either avoiding the inciting activity or bracing herself emotionally. But the unexpected pain was frightening. Catherine got chest pain while reaching up to take a can off her kitchen shelf, and was so distraught, she never did eat the lunch she had been about to prepare. She woke up at four A.M. one day, got up to go to the bathroom, and got chest pain on the way. She sat in the bathroom for half an hour, long after the pain had subsided, anxious that the return trip would result in a repeat performance.

When Saturday rolled around and Jennifer called to arrange their evening out, Catherine had to say she didn't feel like going. Jennifer was alarmed. "Why not? What's the matter?" she asked suspiciously.

"Oh, nothing much. I'm just tired," Catherine answered, trying to suggest that it was just a case of her usual fatigue, only a little more intense.

"But I'll pick you up in my car. I can drop you off at the restaurant before I park. You don't need any energy."

"I just don't feel like it. I've been going to bed very early. I start getting ready at seven and turn in at eight."

Jennifer knew her mother too well to be satisfied with this explanation. "Do you have the flu or something?"

"No, nothing like that."

"So it must be your heart." At least so far, heart problems had been the only major health issue to afflict Catherine. "Are you short of breath?"

"My breathing's not bad."

"What do you mean, not bad? Is it okay or isn't it?"

"It's okay except—except when the pain starts."

"What pain? What do you mean?"

"The chest pains," Catherine finally admitted. "They're back."

Jennifer took a day off from work and brought her mother to see her cardiologist. He looked somber as he studied Catherine Endicott's electrocardiogram, taken during a brief episode of chest pain she fortuitously developed as she climbed onto the examining table. "It's ischemic all right." He looked up. "It's angina."

"We knew that," Jennifer barked. "We're here to figure out what to do about it."

The cardiologist looked over the top of his reading glasses at the two of them. Catherine, dignified, calm, her neatly buttoned blouse concealing a heart that was in tough shape. Jennifer, abrasive, mannish, her power suit concealing a caring daughter who was afraid she was about to lose her mother.

"Well, there's bypass surgery," the cardiologist began.

"I've already said no to that."

"But things are different now, Mom."

"Yes and no. I assume the risk of stroke during surgery is, if anything, higher now than it was a couple of years ago. I'm a worse operative risk because I'm older. What else do you have in mind, Doctor?"

"I could change your medications around a little. There isn't much maneuvering room, since you're already on all the heart medications we have. All I can do is to increase the dose and hope your blood pressure doesn't get too low."

"Let's try it."

The cardiologist was skeptical. "I think we should bring you into the hospital and cool you off with intravenous medication. Then we can see if changes in your oral medications keep things quiet."

"That sounds like a good idea," Jennifer agreed.

Catherine was reluctant. She did not want to go to the hospital. She was afraid a whole team of doctors would try to twist her arm to get her to agree to surgery. But she was frightened of being alone at home, watching the clock, measuring how many minutes elapsed before the pain returned. And the truth was, she was not ready to die. Her refusal of surgery continued to be a rational decision to avoid what she regarded as intolerable potential complications. A procedure without the unacceptably high risks of open heart surgery, a procedure that might keep her going and would get rid of the awful pains—that was another matter. Catherine agreed to hospitalization.

Exactly such a low-risk procedure is what the cardiologist proposed two days later. Blood tests and serial electrocardiograms had demonstrated that Catherine was not having another heart attack. The intravenous medication her doctor had discussed in the office was successful in eradicating the pain, but as soon as it was stopped and she was switched to oral medications, the pains returned. Twice the doctors turned on the magical intravenous drip, only to be unable to keep her pain-free when they turned it off. At that point, Dr. Fields, her cardiologist, met with Catherine and both her daughters to discuss the options.

"We need to do a cardiac catheterization," he said simply.

"I don't want surgery," Catherine reminded him.

"I know that. But the cath will allow us to see if you're a candidate for angioplasty. That's the Roto-Rooter treatment I'm sure you've heard about." He explained that if there were a few short, discrete areas of narrowing responsible for the chest pains, the cardiologist could perform a second procedure, this time threading a special balloon-tipped catheter into the offending blood vessel and squeezing the atherosclerotic plaque onto the walls of the artery. It was not a risk-free procedure: the dye used during the catheterization to outline the passage of blood through the coronary arteries could trigger kidney problems. Catherine knew about those—her husband had died of renal failure. The balloon sometimes momentarily blocked the already narrowed blood vessel entirely, producing pain and perhaps even heart damage. At worst, though this complication was rare, the catheter punctured a coronary artery. Emergency surgery would then be the only way to prevent death.

"I'll do it," Catherine announced, to her daughters' infinite relief. "But no surgery. If they stick the catheter through my blood vessel, that's it." Dr. Fields looked pained. "It's okay. If I die, I promise I won't sue." They all laughed a tense, uncomfortable laugh.

"The interventional cardiologists—the ones who do the procedure—prefer having surgical backup. They don't like feeling that if there's trouble, their hands are tied."

"They don't have to like it, but will they do it?" Dr. Fields nodded. "Well, then, it's settled."

The next morning, Catherine Endicott was wheeled to the cath lab, as the procedure room was known. At 7:00 sharp, the diagnostic catheterization began. At 7:52, it was completed. Catherine was taken to the coronary care unit for observation. At 9:30, the attending cardiologist reviewed her condition and her electrocardiogram, and pronounced the procedure uneventful. Catherine returned to a regular room on the hospital's cardiac floor.

At four P.M., Dr. Fields stopped by to see his patient and inform her of the results of the catheterization. There were profound narrowings in all three major blood vessels supplying the heart. One area of blockage was too extensive to be amenable to angioplasty. One area of blockage was thought to be unrelated to Catherine's symptoms. The third area of narrowing just might be possible to repair.

"So when will you do it?"

Dr. Fields smiled. He liked this feisty lady, who seemed to know what she wanted and what she didn't want. He found her two daughters intimidating, but Catherine was easy to get along with. "How about tomorrow morning? Same time, same place."

Catherine telephoned her daughters with the news. Jennifer was disappointed that she had not been there to interrogate Dr. Fields. Andrea decided she would page Fields and quiz him on the chances of success. "I want to know what makes him so sure this is going to work. What if the trouble is coming from one of the other blockages? How can they tell? If this doesn't work, will they keep taking you to the lab and trying new spots?"

"You can call him if you like," Catherine commented, "but I've made up my mind."

Catherine Endicott's intuition was good: the procedure went as smoothly as the first catheterization. Apart from her heart disease, she was in fairly good physical condition. She had a touch of arthritis—her fingers and knees ached now and then. Her hearing was not as good as it once had been, but otherwise she was fine. Certainly there was a possibility that blood vessels in other parts of her body were narrowed from atherosclerosis as well. The vessels bringing blood to the kidneys, legs, and brain had all been affected in her husband's case, but Catherine had no symptoms to indicate she had any other critically narrowed arteries. Her blood tests gave no hint of impaired kidney function, she never got cramps in her legs when she walked, and she had suffered neither a mini-stroke nor a full-blown one.

The cardiologist who performed the angioplasty was extremely skilled in the subtleties of the procedure. He was technically adept and had a large dose of that nebulous but critical substance known as clinical judgment. What that meant, Dr. Fields had explained to Catherine, was that if he encountered the unexpected, he would be able to figure out what to do. "A good technician can do the procedure when everything goes by the book," he told her. "The problem is when the catheter won't go in the right place, or the patient gets the worst chest pain of his life, or something like that. The doctor has to decide whether to go on or to bail out. Sometimes he has to improvise. Making the right choice—the choice that results in the best outcome for the patient—that's good clinical judgment." In Catherine's case, the procedure was a little tricky, but the doctor used excellent clinical judgment. The last remaining question was whether the angioplasty would prevent further chest pain.

For twenty-four hours after the procedure, Catherine was confined to bed with a weight on her groin to prevent bleeding from the puncture site, the spot at which the catheter had entered her body and been threaded all the way into the heart. After breakfast the following morning, a nurse escorted Catherine from her bed to the bathroom. Gingerly, she reached up to brush her hair, a motion she had learned to associate with chest pain. Nothing happened. She finished in the bathroom and asked if she might walk down the corridor to the nurses' station.

Cautiously, anxiously, Catherine made her way down the hall. Then, more confident, she sped up slightly. Still nothing. She turned around, returned to her room, and sat down in a chair by the window. If she had not been taking medication to decrease the work of her heart, medication that kept her heart rate low, her heart would have been racing from nervousness. Catherine rested a few minutes, and then, overtaken by the urge to see if the feat could be duplicated, she got up for another lap.

When Jennifer came to take her mother home that afternoon, she found her walking down the corridor. Slowly, methodically, her head held high, Catherine Endicott was convincing herself that the angioplasty had worked. Her heart was too damaged from the old heart attack to pump well, so she still tired easily and got short of breath from strenuous exertion. But the debilitating and demoralizing chest pains had vanished. Catherine bought herself a cane, gave up her volunteer job at the library, and got on with her life.

...

Coronary artery disease is the leading cause of death in those over sixty-five. As the story of Catherine Endicott makes clear, it is also a major source of disability.[7] Improvements in medical care (coronary care units, new medications, and treatment of high blood pressure and high cholesterol) as well as lifestyle changes (principally in the realm of diet and exercise) have led to a decline in both the rate of new cases of heart disease each year and the death rate from heart disease.[8] Despite these advances, angina and myocardial infarction remain major health problems, especially for the elderly. Treatment options have expanded considerably, with three principal approaches: medical intervention, surgical intervention, or, midway in terms of invasiveness, procedures such as angioplasty or stent-placement.[9]

Stent-placement is a variant of angioplasty in that it is a procedure designed to open up narrowed blood vessels during a cardiac catheterization. Instead of widening the coronary arteries with a balloon, small stainless steel stents, shaped much like tiny straws, are inserted into the problem area. Stents have the advantage that they are permanent, so they are likely to keep the blood vessel open. However, they work best if there is a single, short area of narrowing. Longer-affected regions may necessitate multiple stents, and blockage can develop between stents.[10]

Catherine Endicott, in whom medical treatment was ineffective and who refused open heart surgery, did extremely well with angioplasty. While clearly an invasive procedure, angioplasty is far less traumatic than the full-blown surgical alternative, a coronary artery bypass graft (CABG). In this type of surgery, the chest is opened, the heart is exposed, the individual is placed on a cardiopulmonary bypass machine so as to empty the heart of blood during the operation, and a vein taken from the leg is grafted onto the diseased artery. Mortality from this surgery, while considered very low, averages 4 percent, compared to less than 1 percent for angioplasty.[11] The recovery from CABG is similarly more complicated and prolonged than from angioplasty. While vigorous individuals, regardless of age, rebound after CABG with remarkable speed (they are often discharged after five days, and frequently go directly home without any inpatient rehabilitation), the frail older person is at risk of developing multiple postoperative complications. He may, for example, get a pneumonia because he fails to take deep breaths after surgery. The antibiotics used to treat the pneumonia may result in colitis, a common complication in debilitated older people. The colitis, in turn, produces weakness that may further impede rehabilitative efforts. Alternatively, the patient may develop a blood clot in the leg, and that clot may travel to the lungs—another potential postoperative complication. Or the patient may get a stress ulcer after surgery. The net result, in many instances, is that the frail person survives surgery such as CABG, but is left at a lower level of functioning from which recovery is slow at best. Less definitive procedures such as angioplasty, by contrast, are associated with a far more uneventful recovery. Discharge is typically within two days and is almost invariably to home.

Angioplasty and stenting are sometimes optimal strategies—just as successful as coronary artery bypass surgery with considerably less risk. In some patients, like Catherine Endicott, in whom a CABG would have been technically preferable, angioplasty can be a satisfactory compromise between the desire to improve quality of life and the dangers of intervention.

Jack Simon

Everyone noticed that although Jack Simon had made enormous progress after his stroke, his right leg remained very weak.

It was sufficiently weak that he could no longer walk and found transferring from his bed to a chair a challenge. What nobody noticed, because it was very subtle, was that ever since the stroke, there was something wrong with Jack's vision. He was not blind, and he did not see double. His vision was not blurred. The problem was that he had a visual-field cut—an entire chunk of his field of vision was missing. What this meant was that he could see everything that was directly in front of him, but objects off to the side he would not even notice unless he turned his head.

The field cut, or hemianopsia, was potentially dangerous because a car could be approaching from the right side as Jack wheeled himself down the street and he would be unaware of it until it was almost on top of him. Fortunately, he could partially compensate for this deficit: his hearing was intact, so he relied on his ears to alert him to an impending arrival. He also learned to compensate consciously—by explicitly attending to what was going on nearby, and by deliberately turning his head. What Jack discovered, however, was that the field cut made reading difficult. Not impossible, but difficult. It wasn't the sort of problem that was helped by a magnifier or a bright light or large-print books. The crux of the matter was that words seemed to jump around on the page. With tremendous discipline and concentration, Jack could read a few pages at a time. He tired easily, and typically had to stop after just a few minutes.

Gradually, almost without being aware of the change, Jack shifted from the paper to the radio as his prime source of news. He discovered that the "talking books" he had once purchased for long car rides were also useful for long winter evenings at home. Fixing things around the house, which had always been his job, became a joint enterprise: his wife read him the directions, got the appropriate tools, and he carried out the repairs—on a tape recorder that malfunctioned or a clock that required resetting—

provided that not much detail work was required. Jack could still read if he had to, he could still watch television, and he could recognize his friends.

A year after the stroke, while living at home with his wife, Jack developed a second problem with his already impaired vision: he began to find that television images were fuzzy. "Something's wrong with the television, Margaret," he announced. Margaret was surprised and commented that she thought the image was perfectly clear. "No, it's not!" Jack snapped. To humor him, Margaret fiddled with the dials, but she could do nothing to improve matters. "Let's try the other television," he suggested. But the small set in their bedroom was just as blurred to him and just as clear to her. Uncharacteristically, Jack began to cry. "I'm falling apart. I can't even see anymore."

Margaret put her arms around him. Jack had put up with so much—he had tolerated the indignity of needing help to bathe and dress, he had endured word-finding difficulties. Each difficulty he had regarded as an obstacle to be overcome. He had been sad, frustrated, frightened that he would never recover enough to live at home with his wife. But he had never *cried*.

"You aren't falling apart," Margaret whispered as she stroked his hair. "Something's the matter with your vision. So we'll go to the eye doctor and see what he can do about it."

"You're always so practical, Margaret," Jack sighed. "But what if, what if . . ." His eyes filled with tears and he could not finish his sentence.

"What if it's another stroke?" His wife completed the thought for him. He nodded. "I don't think it is. I think you've been having trouble for some time. Remember how the light's been bothering your eyes? And how you find that you can read better without your glasses than with them?" Jack nodded again. "I don't think this has anything to do with the old stroke, or that it means a new stroke. Actually, I think I know what the problem is."

"You do?"

"I think you have a cataract in your right eye. Remember Dr. Jeffreys said something about an early cataract when you saw him two years ago? We were supposed to go back last year, but you had the stroke, so we forgot about it." Margaret smiled, pleased with her diagnosis.

"You're brilliant," Jack told her proudly.

"My friend Betsy had a cataract and she had exactly the same symptoms. When it really started to bother her, she had surgery and had a lens implant. She's fine now."

Jack looked apprehensive again. "But would they operate on me? I'm eighty-one and I've had a stroke."

"I don't see why not. The rest of you is in working order."

Jack became teary-eyed again. He did not feel that his other parts were functioning very well—his legs would not support him, his arm did not allow him to write clearly. What Margaret meant was that the fundamentals were operational: his heart, his lungs, and, above all, his mind. Moreover, his disabilities had not prevented him from living at home, socializing with friends and family, and remaining in touch with his clients—the middle-aged executives whom he had helped find new jobs after they lost their old ones.

During the two weeks before his eye doctor appointment, Jack was alternately confident and terrified. When he was confident, he believed his wife's diagnosis, he was certain there was an easy fix for his problem, and he even rationalized that the blurred vision wasn't such a big deal, so it wouldn't matter if nothing could be done. On other days, he was equally convinced that his wife was mistaken and that he had had a new stroke. Not only did he believe his visual difficulty was uncorrectable, but he was certain he was destined to have a relentless series of strokes, each of which would leave him appreciably more debilitated and dependent. At times, Jack was so distraught by his beliefs and so certain of his prognosis that he wanted to cancel the ophthalmology appointment. He would rather live with a faint ray of hope than with the certainty of gloom he was sure the appointment would bring.

Margaret practically had to drag him to the doctor. Since getting to the office was no mean feat—she had to arrange for a chair car to transport both him and his wheelchair because he had not mastered the art of getting in and out of a regular car—taking him when he was reluctant to go was almost impossible. But Margaret prevailed, insisting over his protests, and the two of them found themselves in Dr. Jeffreys's office.

After a half-hour wait, Margaret wheeled her husband in to see Dr. Jeffreys. The verdict was delivered swiftly. Jack had a mature cataract in his right eye. It could easily be removed with a simple operation, and he would go home with a new plastic lens implanted in its stead. The odds were that his vision would be restored, though very occasionally there was a complication that made matters worse rather than better. In some cases, an unsuspected additional abnormality was found, such as damage to the retina of the eye, which persisted after removal of the cataract. In those instances, the operation was a technical success, but vision was not improved. It was all very routine, Dr. Jeffreys assured the couple. His schedule was full, so the earliest he could book the operation was in a month.

That month was a nightmare for the Simons. Margaret was surprised: she had expected that Jack would calm down once a plan was in place. She thought he would be reassured by the diagnosis, comforted by how commonplace cataracts were. After fifty-five years of marriage, Jack was still not entirely predictable. Instead of eagerly awaiting his cataract surgery, he became progressively more despondent. When he could not make out the headlines in *The Boston Globe,* he canceled his subscription. When he realized his wife had bought regular hamburger meat instead of the extra-lean variety that he preferred, he fumed and fretted and insisted on throwing out the meat. When Margaret went out to a movie with friends, she returned to find Jack sitting in his wheelchair in the dark, staring straight ahead. He worried that the operation would be a failure, that he would end up blind in one eye. He began to fantasize that the surgery would somehow provoke a new stroke.

His moodiness, his fears, his irrationality, were all triggered by a growing conviction that his life was over. He would, he was sure, become totally dependent on his wife. He would lose the ability to do any of the things that gave him pleasure—advising his clients, socializing with his family. Jack was prepared to die. The only problem was that he was not terminally ill. He might linger in his current state for years.

Margaret toyed with bringing Jack to a psychiatrist, but she could not imagine persuading him to go voluntarily. She seriously considered lacing his coffee with antidepressants, "borrowed" from one of her friends, but realized she would be mortified if he developed side effects. She imagined herself convicted of prescribing without a medical license, languishing in jail. On balance, she concluded that the best strategy was to tough it out until after the surgery.

Two days after the operation, Jack Simon was transformed. His vision was dramatically improved. It would be a couple of months before he could be refracted for new glasses, but having gone through the procedure and discovering that he really would regain useful sight was enough to boost his spirits. He was scarcely bothered by the fact that he still could not read for more than a few minutes at a time because the words jumped around on the page. His right leg weakness did not seem to disturb him at all, now that his fears of a second stroke had not been realized.

The Simons went out for dinner to celebrate Jack's eighty-second birthday. Jack ordered a selection that carried the American Heart Association "healthy heart" approval. "I'm planning to be around for another ten years, so I want to stay fit," he explained to the waiter.

"To the next decade," Margaret said as they clinked wineglasses. They had chosen a full-bodied red wine, alleged to decrease the risk of heart attacks when consumed in moderation.

Cataracts are the seventh most common chronic condition reported by older Americans, affecting nearly one-fifth of all people over sixty-five. A cataract is simply an opacification of the normally transparent lens of the eye, which is a crystalline structure that is two-thirds water and one-third protein. With age, the water content of the lens tends to decrease and changes in the protein component develop, causing loss of transparency.[12]

Treatment of cataracts is exclusively surgical: there is no pill that cures cataracts. Fortunately, the surgical techniques are now very sophisticated. Cataract surgery, which involves removal of the lens, used to be an inpatient procedure, associated with a lengthy period of recuperation. Moreover, once the natural lens was gone, individuals had to wear extremely thick glasses. Not only were these glasses unattractive but they distorted visual images, magnifying them as much as 25 percent. As contact lenses became widely accepted, patients could be fitted with contacts instead of glasses. The heavy, unsightly spectacles were replaced by lenses that magnified only 1 percent. Many older individuals, however, lacked the dexterity necessary to use contact lenses. The great breakthrough in cataract surgery was the development of the lens implant. At the time of surgery, an artificial lens is inserted to replace the cloudy, poorly functioning original. The technique has been modified so that the entire procedure is done on an outpatient basis, using local anesthesia. Patients do have to wear a patch for a couple of days and need to use special drops for a time, so they may need some assistance for a week or two after the operation.

The results of cataract surgery are excellent, with 95 percent of those patients who have no significant other eye diseases achieving 20/40 vision. Complications, including bleeding into the eye and infection, occur in fewer than 5 percent of patients. In a small number of people, the retina, which was previously hidden from the eye doctor's view by the cloudy lens, turns out to be diseased as well. In those patients, cataract surgery, while not harmful, proves to be useless.

Cataracts are removed once vision is so impaired that it interferes with functioning. The function in question can be work-related, or it can be reading or watching television. As cataracts "mature," as the lens becomes cloudier, vision is further impaired. Early or immature cataracts are not generally operated on: the rate of progression is typically quite slow and varies from person to person. There is no fixed time at which a cataract must be taken out. Indeed, the only consequence of leaving a cataract in place is its effect on vision. Since there is no danger from leaving a cataract in, it follows that cataracts should be left alone if visual improvement is unlikely to have any meaningful effect on performance. Someone with good vision in one eye and a cataract in the other has no reason to have surgery unless having two working eyes would make a measurable difference in his life—if the added depth perception could prevent falls or car accidents or permit reading. A cognitively impaired individual who is no longer able to understand the written word should not undergo surgery in the vain hope that if his vision were better he could read—the problem is in the brain, not the eye. However, a person with dementia who used to enjoy watching television and no longer does so and who claims she's no longer interested might in fact benefit from surgery: she may have given up watching because the screen was blurred but she had been unable to understand or articulate the real reason for her professed disinterest. Cataract surgery in this setting can help the patient derive satisfaction from an otherwise tedious and empty life.

Medicare spends more than 3 billion dollars per year on cataract surgery for older people.[13] It is the most common surgical procedure performed in the elderly. Even those in their nineties and above can benefit from surgery. Risks of systemic complications such as heart attacks are minuscule. Perhaps the most serious and underestimated risk is the development of delirium—transient confusion associated with surgery—but this is a risk worth taking if the benefit, as with Jack Simon, is a new lease on life.

Leyla Keribar

Valerie brought her mother to my office because her arthritis and her Parkinson's disease were worse—she had trouble walking and the tremor was so bad that she had spilled hot soup on herself twice in one week and could hardly play the piano. She was refusing to take her blood-pressure medication because she said it made her dizzy. And her hip hurt her so badly when she moved it that she screamed out in pain.

I asked which problem bothered her the most, and Leyla just shook her head. "I can't stand it anymore. It's awful."

Valerie was almost as desperate as her mother. "I can't do anything to help. I've tried giving her a massage. I bought herbal rheumatism medication because Tylenol didn't work. I told her to stop eating soup since she spills it, and she insists that the only thing that could conceivably cure her is chicken soup." Valerie was on the verge of tears. "She's been calling in the middle of the night—every night for the last week. It's like having a newborn baby in the house." There was an edge to Valerie's voice that I had never heard before.

"I can't help it," Leyla responded indignantly. "I'm as quiet as I can be. You're a light sleeper."

"Newborn babies can't help it either," Valerie snapped. "They wake up. They're hungry. They cry. You wake up with pain. You call out." She softened her tone. "Of course you can't help it. Of course you don't mean to bother me. But I can't help hearing you. And I care that you're hurting. I want to help you. I can't take it anymore either."

Both women were crying now. I waited a moment. "This is a problem I should be able to do something about." Leyla looked at me skeptically. Valerie was cautiously optimistic. "But first let me examine you."

Step one of the examination was watching Leyla get out of a chair. She had to use her arms to push off the sides of her seat. I doubted that she would have been able to extricate herself from a chair without side arms. She would have been held captive by a soft sofa. She made her way to the examining room, walking very slowly. She winced as, with my help, she climbed onto the examining table. I bent her hips one at a time and heard the characteristic grinding sound of bone rubbing against bone when I manipulated her right hip. She grimaced. I asked her to bend her right leg, first at the hip, then at the knee. She stopped after 20 or 30 degrees of flexion—the pain was too great to continue. The left leg was somewhat better: she could move it more readily, farther, and with less discomfort. I palpated her joints: both knees, her wrists, the small joints of her hands. Leyla Keribar appeared to have classic degenerative joint disease, or osteoarthritis, the

wear-and-tear arthritis of aging. There was little or no inflammation of the joints—no swelling, no redness, no warm tender
spots. The joints were simply wearing away, the normal lubricating fluid essentially gone.

I escorted Leyla back to my office, where her daughter was
waiting. She was composed now, and had used the few minutes
alone to dry her tears and powder her face.

"We have a few options," I began. "First, there is medication.
Let's review what you have already tried." She had started with
Tylenol, using as much as two extra-strength capsules every four
hours, with minimal benefit. I had prescribed several different
nonsteroidal anti-inflammatory medications, which she had tried
in maximal doses, again with little effect. The nonsteroidals had
also made her nauseated, so she had stopped after a few days. She
had been lucky that she had not developed a full-blown ulcer or
gastritis, erosions of the lining of the stomach that occur in many
elderly patients on these drugs.[14] I had substituted a new pain
medication, Ultram, which had helped a little, but only at the
highest dose recommended, a dose that also caused Leyla to
become confused and disoriented. "You haven't taken either
Tylenol with codeine or Percocet," I observed.

"I don't want any addicting drugs," Leyla asserted. We talked
about that for a while. Many patients are unreasonably frightened
of using narcotic analgesics—pain medications related to morphine. They fear dependence on the drug even more than the
dependency from their pain. I argued with Leyla: most patients
who take narcotics do not become addicted. If she did develop
tolerance—needing a higher dose to achieve the same effect—I
would prescribe a higher dose. In the event that she actually
became dependent, it would be a worthwhile price to pay to be
relieved of her pain. "You aren't going to become a junkie," I
pointed out. "You aren't going to mug people in the street to get
the money for a fix."

Valerie burst out laughing. The image of her mother holding up passersby was outrageous. Even if her mobility were not limited by pain, even if it were not limited by her parkinsonian rigidity, violence was out of character. "I can see you now, Mom, shuffling down the street, raising your cane, calling out politely in your velvety Turko-French accent, 'Would you please hand over your wallet?'"

We all smiled, but Leyla still did not like the sound of taking narcotics. "Isn't there anything else?"

"There is the surgical option," I replied. "Orthopedic surgeons can replace a hip that has been worn away by arthritis with a new, artificial hip. It's a great operation. It eliminates pain, the new joint works very well, and it lasts for years. Many years. You're seventy-nine? It should last the rest of your life."

Leyla was skeptical. She had heard of hip surgery after fractures, but a hip replacement for arthritis? I assured her that it was a fairly routine procedure. "Let me think about it," was all I could get from her.

"But in the meantime," her daughter chimed in, "how about if you get a prescription for Tylenol with codeine so you at least have something when the pain is very bad."

I agreed. "At least take one before you go to bed, so perhaps you will both get a good night's sleep," I suggested, handing Leyla the prescription. She turned it over to Valerie. "And call me in a few days to let me know how you're doing."

It was Valerie who called. "Mom is a little better. She is taking the new pill at night, and she manages to sleep four or five hours straight."

"How about if she takes another one when she wakes up in the middle of the night?"

"She won't do it. She tried it once, and she felt sleepy the entire next day."

"What about during the day? How bad is the daytime pain?"

"Pretty bad. She sits most of the day and doesn't do anything so as to avoid moving her hip. She's bored and angry. I'm afraid she's getting depressed again."

"Maybe taking two pills just four hours apart was too much for her. Perhaps one at bedtime, one in the morning, and an extra in the early afternoon if she needs it." Valerie was doubtful her mother would be willing to "take so much dope," but she promised to ask her to. She also said they would talk more about surgery.

Two weeks later, Leyla Keribar and her daughter were back in my office. "I can't take that codeine," Leyla announced. "It makes me constipated and sick to my stomach." I launched into my lecture about constipation, kicking myself for not having made certain at the outset that she took prune juice or laxatives along with the codeine. Leyla was not interested. "I've decided to see an orthopedist. I've made up my mind. I don't care if I die—I can't live like this."

I shifted gears and broached the subject of surgical risk. "You won't die," I told her. "Or at least it's very unlikely. The risk is not so much that you could die as that you could have very unpleasant but nonlethal complications. After hip surgery, for instance, there is a risk of developing a blood clot in the leg, and sometimes those clots travel to the lungs. With any major operation," I went on, "there is a risk of cardiac complications. You've had high blood pressure, though it is well controlled with medications right now, and as far as we know, your heart is in pretty good shape." I decided not to go into more detail about the risks at that point. It was, after all, progress for Leyla even to consider an operation. I did not want to discourage her. I did want her to understand that a hip replacement, while a potentially liberating operation, had its downside. And all too frequently, surgeons focused only on mortality when discussing risk, rather than on the far more debilitating and, to my patients, disconcerting threat of disability.

Leyla Keribar was a very determined woman. When she lived in Turkey, she had been determined to enable her daughter to escape the increasingly oppressive political environment. She had corresponded with friends abroad and learned of a fledgling American university that was developing a reputation for high-quality research. With perseverance, she managed to gather the necessary materials for her daughter to apply for a graduate fellowship. The university, seeking talented students and forced to compete with better-known institutions for the cream of the crop, was intrigued by this applicant from a country that was partly in Europe and partly in Asia. Her letters of recommendation were very strong, and her grades—whatever they meant—were excellent. The school took a chance, and Leyla said farewell to her only child. For five years they corresponded weekly but never heard each other's voice, let alone embraced one another. Then, finding Turkey intolerable and longing desperately to see Valerie, Leyla and her husband obtained a tourist visa to come to the United States.

They never returned to their native land. They left behind their home, their possessions, and their friends to start a new life in America.

Moving to a new country at age sixty was far more difficult than Leyla had anticipated. Even though he was a lawyer, her husband was unemployable in a country with a totally different legal system. She, despite her prodigious linguistic talent, which enabled her to communicate very well, had no marketable skills. But Leyla was a supremely determined woman: once she had decided to uproot herself, she did whatever it took to make a new life. Her attitude to the proposed hip surgery was similar. Once she decided this was the optimal course, there was no deviating from the chosen path. She took the initiative to schedule the orthopedic appointment herself instead of passively turning the planning or decision-making responsibility to her daughter.

Leyla's conviction that she was doing the right thing helped get her through the surgery and then the three weeks at a rehabilitation hospital. She worked hard in physical therapy—exercising, walking, and then falling into an exhausted sleep each night. When I saw her for follow-up in my office, both she and her daughter looked as though they were back from a long, leisurely vacation. For Valerie, it had been a holiday, or at least respite from the sleepless nights and tension-filled days. For Leyla, the vacation had been more like a hectic guided tour rather than a stay at a luxury resort, but she was exhilarated by her progress. "I cooked dinner last night," she told me proudly. "For the whole family: Valerie and George and the boys. I don't think I made quite enough, though. Adolescent boys have voracious appetites."

"You made plenty, Mom," Valerie defended her. "They had to save room for the lime custard pie. And after months of my cooking, they were delighted to have such a delicious meal." She turned to me. "Mom is an astonishing cook. Somehow she never taught me her secrets."

I was glad to see the two of them sparring again, playfully. The angry edge was gone from Valerie's voice. "Did you have any trouble maneuvering around the kitchen?" I asked, changing the subject.

"No pain. Not a twinge. But I'm slow and I'm stiff." I tested her motor function, her gait. Now that pain was not limiting her, I could see the extent of her rigidity. It was mild, but conspicuous enough to get in the way of her doing all she wanted to. The time had come, I thought, to increase the dose of her Sinemet, the medication that partially replaced the neurotransmitter dopamine, which was lacking in Parkinson's disease. Now that the osteoarthritis pain was under control, we could take the next small step in improving Leyla's overall condition.

Antiparkinsonian medications do not cure Parkinson's disease. They rarely obliterate the symptoms, though they decrease them enough to make an appreciable difference in life. The underlying disease progresses, however, and after a few years, even with dosage adjustments, the medications are not very effective. Addition of other medications that work in a slightly different way to compensate for the state of dopamine deficiency are of modest benefit. Ultimately, parkinsonian patients cannot walk and are unable to feed themselves. Leyla had a long way to go before reaching that point. In the meantime, I would continue to strive to fix the reversible components of her chronic illnesses, and to ameliorate the irreversible components.

When older people are asked to list the medical problems that interfere most with their lives, arthritis always comes out as number one.[15] And by far the most common form of arthritis is osteoarthritis, or degenerative joint disease.

Osteoarthritis can affect many different joints, with the hips and the knees as its major targets. This kind of arthritis creates two problems: pain and limitation of function. To some extent, the two are related—pain is one of the causes of decreased range of motion, hence mobility. In addition, the wearing away of the joint itself, with loss of its normal lubricating fluid, prevents the joint from doing what it is designed for—bending. Medication can be helpful in osteoarthritis, particularly pain medication such as acetaminophen or aspirin. Many people get relief from nonsteroidal anti-inflammatory medication (such as ibuprofen). This type of medication, however, can cause gastrointestinal bleeding, kidney abnormalities, and confusion, so it is far from ideal. In fact, at least one study in which patients were given either Tylenol (acetominophen) or Motrin (ibuprofen) but did not know which they were getting found no difference between them in effectiveness.[16]

Approximately 120,000 total hip replacements are performed each year in the United States, two-thirds of that number in people over age sixty-five. If a patient has X-ray evidence of joint damage and moderate to severe persistent pain or disability unrelieved by medication or physical therapy, he or she is a candidate for surgery.[17] Until recently, the surgery sometimes had to be redone because the prosthesis loosened and no longer worked properly. With the introduction of new kinds of cement and prostheses made of new material (commonly an alloy of cobalt and titanium), loosening has become very rare. Studies of patients undergoing the procedure for arthritis find that it produces an immediate substantial decrease in pain, better function, and improved health-related quality of life.

Hip fracture is another reason for a total hip replacement in the elderly. While certain types of fracture can be treated with internal fixation, using one or more screws, other types are best treated with a total hip replacement. This is often the case in older people with a displaced fracture. Whether the surgery is performed because of a fracture or osteoarthritis, surgical complications have been decreased because of the use of antibiotics to prevent infection and anticoagulants to avoid postoperative blood clots. Rehabilitation is started promptly—usually the day after surgery—and patients are transferred to a setting in which they can receive vigorous physical therapy.

The interventions described in this chapter—Ben Frank's hearing aid, Catherine Endicott's angioplasty, Jack Simon's cataract surgery, and Leyla Keribar's hip replacement—are not cures for frailty. Yet, they all had a profoundly positive impact on quality of life. When his hearing was very impaired, Ben became isolated and depressed, scarcely interacting with his family and seldom going out. Once he accepted his deficit and adjusted to a hearing aid, he ventured out of his apartment, making a friend, enjoying the movies. Catherine was incapacitated by her angina: unable to cook or clean or go out, either because the exertion produced chest pain and shortness of breath or because of the equally disabling fear that those activities would lead to symptoms. Once she underwent a procedure to open up the clogged arteries feeding her heart, the pain vanished, and with it, much of her anxiety. She was able to live independently again—her activities circumscribed, her adventurousness diminished, but her spirit reinvigorated. Jack Simon was similarly devastated by his visual loss, coming as it did on top of his already impaired vision and his physical weakness. As with Catherine, the human inclination to think ahead, to try to imagine the future, had a deleterious effect on Jack. He worried that he would lose his sight altogether. A visit to his ophthalmologist reassured him somewhat, but the ultimate reassurance stemmed from successful cataract surgery. Leyla Keribar's hip replacement almost certainly slowed the progression of her frailty. Once her mobility improved, thanks to the surgery, her overall functioning became far less tenuous.

It is no accident that several of the interventions that made such a difference in overall functioning were surgical. Operating on a frail person who has limited organ reserve can be a perilous undertaking, but the kinds of operations that Jack and Leyla underwent were relatively minor. Cataract surgery is done on an ambulatory basis—gone are the days of overnight hospital stays with their attendant confusion and disruption. Local anesthesia is used for cataract surgery, and spinal anesthesia is commonly used for hip surgery, thus avoiding the systemic effects of general anesthesia.

As technology advances, physicians can increasingly substitute minimally invasive procedures for major surgery. Sometimes the surgical approach is statistically preferable—that is, it is more likely to be effective over the long run. For an eighty-five-year-old, the long run may be of little consequence. In other cases, technology has simply rendered the old form of treatment obsolete. Laparoscopic cholecystectomy, for instance, is rapidly replacing traditional gallbladder surgery. In this approach, the surgeon makes a tiny incision in the abdomen, and introduces a special tube through which the entire operation is conducted. Only when the new approach is technically impossible, typically due to prior surgery, does it make sense to open up the abdomen with a six-inch incision instead. Likewise, polyps are commonly removed through a colonoscope rather than by cutting open the abdomen and excising a portion of the colon.

Fixing the fixable aspect of frailty does not always necessitate a surgical or quasi-surgical intervention. Medication can play an important role, as with antidepressants, or with Leyla Keribar's Parkinson's medication. Both medicines and surgery entail risk, though with medications, most of the side effects are readily reversible. The adverse reactions from medications range from acute confusion to falls, with constipation, nausea, and headache as other frequently reported side effects. When pills do not bring problems in their wake, they have the potential to alleviate frailty. Sinemet cured neither Leyla's Parkinson's nor her frailty, but it decreased her stiffness and made it easier for her to start moving. Sinemet would have had the same neurologic effect had Parkinson's been Leyla's only problem, but it had a larger functional effect since the combination of osteoarthritis and Parkinson's had left Leyla severely limited.

Antidepressants are another class of drug that can be critical for the frail. While Ben Frank suffered an adverse reaction from the antidepressant nortriptyline, developing urinary retention, Leyla Keribar would later derive benefit from the antidepressant Prozac. Whether frail individuals become depressed as a reaction to their increasing disability and dependence or they develop depression on top of and separate from their other medical problems, depressive symptoms sap them of needed emotional energy. Depression can deprive the frail of the will necessary to cope with their physical condition. Depression may also interact with other medical problems: the person who does not eat and drink enough becomes dehydrated, which in turn can trigger a cycle of weakness, falls, and fractures—leading to worsening frailty. Alternatively, apathy and loss of interest in life can lead to a very sedentary existence, which can result in a blood clot, and hence further inactivity and disability. Treatment of depression, usually by medications, sometimes with psychotherapy, or, as in Ben Frank's case, simply by fixing his hearing, can prevent a cascade of untoward events.

Fixing the fixable part is crucial for the frail person, not because of its consequences for particular organ systems, nor for its effects on longevity, but rather because it results in improvement in function. Although diseases of particular organs such as the heart or lungs or kidneys can certainly affect functioning, the conditions that are often most important to attend to—and those most likely to be neglected by nongeriatrically oriented physicians—are those involving the senses. Improving the ability to hear and see is critical. Attending to gait and balance is extremely important. Functioning, or the ability to carry out those activities essential to maintaining integrity as a human being, is the focus of geriatrics. Frailty, the heart of which is diminished functioning, is the quintessential geriatric condition. Moderating the effects of frailty is what geriatric medicine is all about.

CHAPTER 3

The Moves Make the Man

My natural inclination, as a physician, is to look for medical solutions to the problems posed by frailty. The incontrovertible benefits of interventions such as cataract surgery, hearing aids, and antidepressant medications testify to the prominent role medicine can play in ameliorating frailty. But frailty implies problems with bathing and dressing, or problems with shopping and cleaning. Coming to terms with frailty means finding a way to get help in these areas. Whether the many needs of the frail elder are effectively met depends on the suitability of his or her *environment*.

By environment, I mean both the physical surroundings and the social milieu. The typical old person has not bargained for her "golden years" to be marked by frailty. She, in all likelihood, is accustomed to taking autonomy, independence, and good health for granted. Not only does she personally place a premium on independence, but she also lives in a society that devalues those who are dependent. Coping with frailty involves more than pills, procedures, and assistive devices: it involves the entire environment.

As Ben Frank, Catherine Endicott, Jack Simon, and Leyla Keribar entered the realm of frailty, they discovered that the homes they were living in were not perfectly suited to their needs. Stairs were suddenly too difficult to climb; cluttered rooms were a hazard if vision was impaired or balance was poor. The family house was too big—too large to clean, too expensive to maintain. Adaptations were necessary, either in the form of physical modifications or in the hiring of personal assistants. In some cases, it made more sense to move out than to renovate and hire helpers. All except Jack, who lived with his wife, struggled with loneliness: Ben and Catherine each lived alone, though they were in close touch with their children; Leyla lived under the same roof as her daughter and son-in-law, but they worked during the day, leaving her alone with her anxiety. Although Jack was not lonely, he was acutely aware of his dependence on his wife. He recognized that if she developed a problem, he would be lost. Moreover, he worried that his wife felt trapped, unable to go anywhere or do anything without first providing for his safety.

The twin themes of loneliness and physical dependence led all four to make changes in their living situations. Fortunately, they lived in a time and place that offered them a panoply of choices: assisted living, continuing-care retirement communities, nursing homes, and community-based long-term care. They had sufficient financial resources and familial support to explore and ultimately select a good option. Their friends were not always so lucky. They would all have benefited from knowing in advance about their choices.

Ben Frank

When her father returned home after his third hospitalization for heart failure, Susan told me angrily that he was weak from having been essentially on bed rest during his entire hospital stay. "If he fell when he wasn't weak, he's certainly going to fall now that he can barely get out of a chair! I don't see how they could send him home like that."

Since hospital payments from Medicare (the federal insurance program covering acute medical care for the elderly) are determined by the patient's diagnosis, hospitals have an incentive to discharge patients "quicker and sicker." Length of stay in the hospital has fallen dramatically and many families feel their relatives are being discharged prematurely.[1]

I asked what kind of assistance had been arranged for him.

"Oh, they told me he would have plenty of 'services.' Actually, he has a visiting nurse who came twice this week to check his blood pressure. The blood pressure was fine, so she'll only come once next week. She spent at most fifteen minutes with Dad, and most of that she spent 'documenting.' That's jargon for writing things down, I learned. Dad estimated she made eye contact with him for no more than five minutes. Tops."

"What about physical therapy?"

"He has a physical therapist. A very nice young man—I met him when I went to check up on my father. He came twice."

"And what did he say about your father's condition?"

"He thinks he should be in a rehab hospital. I asked about getting him into one, and I was told that it's very hard to do from home. You pretty much have to be in a hospital. I said Dad had just been in the hospital, but he told me it was too late."

Medicare has a "three-day rule," which requires that patients be in an acute-care hospital for seventy-two hours in order to be eligible for either a rehabilitation hospital or skilled-nursing facility benefits.

"Maybe he should be in a nursing home. Just short-term. Lots of nursing home stays are temporary. They're basically a low-key alternative to the rehab hospital. Many people find the intensive pace of inpatient rehab too much—they have rules, too, and their main one is the two-hour rule. Medicare will reimburse only if the patient receives a minimum of two hours a day of skilled physical therapy, occupational therapy, or speech therapy. They usually have to qualify for at least two different forms of therapy as well."

Susan was not pleased with this suggestion. "Dad wants to stay home."

"Of course he would prefer to stay home. But being in a nursing home for a little while is like being in the hospital. You'd rather not be there, but sometimes it's necessary."

Susan did not think that being in a nursing home was at all like being in a hospital. To her, and no doubt to her father, a hospital was a place where you got help, where technology and professional expertise, and sometimes plain human decency, combined to make sick people well. A nursing home, by contrast, she regarded as a warehouse for storing society's discards, those too feeble and too poor to survive on their own.

I didn't hear from Susan for the next three weeks. We were both busy people who moved in different worlds. I had my work and my family; she had her job as a book designer, many hobbies, and a full social life. Reminded of our longstanding relationship by an invitation to attend our college reunion, we got together for lunch.

"My dad's been doing all right," Susan began. Any anger over my implication that perhaps he should be in a nursing home was gone. Susan was simply relieved that he was managing at home.

"His doctor in New York thought he needed a nursing home and so did the physical therapist and the visiting nurse. Even I thought he probably needed a nursing home," Susan admitted. "We've just been really lucky. I found a marvelous woman to take care of Dad. She works six hours a day, five days a week. She cooks, she cleans, and she's company. Her favorite song is 'You are my sunshine, my only sunshine.' She gets Dad to smile."

"That's wonderful!" Did I dare ask about weekends?

Susan read my mind. "For a while we had someone coming weekends, too—Josie. Josie was loud and not very thorough. Dad didn't especially care for her. He seemed to be managing, so we let her go. It's just as well, because this is costing a fortune. Dad's living on social security and a small pension from his job. He does have the life insurance from Mom. My brother and I always said there was no point in their having life insurance once we were grown up, but they didn't listen to us. Anyway, it came in handy. Dad's been using the money from Mom's life insurance to pay for Carmela. I don't know what he's going to do when it runs out."

Financing home care is no trivial matter. Medicare has only very limited home-care benefits. A patient with an acute medical problem—for example, someone recently discharged from the hospital, recovering from an infection or a heart attack—is eligible to have a visiting nurse come out to the home. Usually the visits are once or twice a week, though more frequent if the nurse needs to change a dressing or draw blood on a regular basis. Nursing visits are usually brief in duration (rarely more than half an hour), and are discontinued once the patient is deemed medically stable. Similarly, other skilled medical personnel, such as a physical therapist (to work on gait and balance, as in Ben Frank's case) or an occupational therapist (to do upper-extremity exercises or to work on retraining patients in how to dress or bathe themselves), are paid for by Medicare in the short term. In general, Medicare covers those services that are "medical" in a very narrow sense. Paradoxically, given that Medicare principally provides care for the elderly, the program is not designed to address chronic illness in general or frailty in particular. Medicare reimburses for care given for an acute illness, but not, with rare exceptions, for ongoing monitoring of chronic problems. There seems to be little recognition that failure to monitor may result in an acute flare of a chronic problem, perhaps necessitating hospitalization. The Medicare program also does not take into consideration that even though an older person may have no single problem that warrants skilled care, the presence of multiple interacting disorders may demand professional treatment. With the Balanced Budget Act of 1997, coverage for home care is even more restricted than previously.[2]

By contrast, Medicaid, the combined federal and state health-insurance program for the poor, construes medical needs in a broader sense. It pays for nursing home care, for instance, even though most of the care provided in a nursing home is not skilled professional care, but rather assistance with the fundamentals of daily life, provided by nursing aides. Medicaid similarly allows for much more in the way of chronic maintenance in the home setting. It will pay for a homemaker (someone to do housework) and a home health aide (someone to provide personal care, such as bathing) for a frail, homebound elder, even if he has not just been discharged from a hospital. The extent of such services, however, is limited, and varies from state to state.[3]

The result of the limitations on publicly funded home health care is that many older people either pay privately for care or enter a nursing home. Once an individual requires the level of care offered by a nursing home, Medicaid will pay in full—assuming the person has depleted virtually all his savings and other resources, such as pension money or personal property. Medicare, parenthetically, pays for one hundred days of nursing-home care per year at most, and then only if the person needs extensive skilled care. To stay at home, people need to pay out of their own pockets for care. Someone who needs an attendant eight hours a day, seven days a week, may easily have to pay $850 per week, or more than $44,000 per year. Live-in help is somewhat less expensive, since room and board are included. This can be a wonderful arrangement for a person with sufficient space if he can find the right person who does not mind being on call for nighttime problems.

For Ben Frank, whose home was a small two-bedroom apartment, live-in help would have been difficult. Even when his daughter, Susan, came for a weekend, she found it awkward to stay in Ben's apartment. They had to share a bathroom, which was not easy because he was taking diuretics and often had to get to the bathroom in a hurry. Ben was lucky in that he found—or, rather, Susan found, working through a home-care agency—a woman he got along with who was willing to work from nine, after she dropped her children off at school, until three, when she picked them up. Carmela was home health aide, homemaker, and companion combined. A virtue of a private arrangement is that the employee does not have to abide by strict regulations delimiting her responsibilities. Carmela, for instance, felt perfectly comfortable giving Ben his medications. He could probably have managed on his own, since he did not take many pills and his memory was good. His problem was that he didn't *like* taking pills, particularly the diuretic, so sometimes he postponed and postponed until he had skipped the pills for a couple of days.

Technically, only a licensed nurse was allowed to administer medication, though an aide could remind her charge to take his pills. Carmela found that the easiest approach was to hand Ben all his medicines and a glass of juice to take them with along with his lunch. It was efficient, he didn't object, and she thought the idea that she might not be "allowed" to pour out his pills was preposterous.

One of the many remarkable consequences of Carmela's arrival was that Ben stopped falling. Even though she was with him only part of the day, and even though he was on his own over the weekend, he generally did better after she started working for him. Perhaps it was because he ate better—he put on five pounds in the month after she started cooking for him, and the gain was not due to fluid retention. Perhaps it was because he slept better at night, without requiring sleeping pills or antidepressants. He began to venture out on the weekends, resuming his former ritual Saturday visit to the corner store and regularly stopping by to visit his neighbors. Perhaps he stopped falling because his mood improved.

When he lived alone without help, Ben had been consumed with anxiety about falling. The first fall had been traumatic—after the episode in which he had been on the floor for an extended period, he had never been quite the same. Though he rarely articulated his fears, he did indicate to his family that he wanted desperately to avoid entering a nursing home, and he had seen enough people carted off to an institution for their own safety after a fall to be worried about this prospect.

Nursing homes can be far more tolerable than many people expect. The horror stories of abuse or insufficient staffing, of overmedication and understimulation, while not entirely past history, are far rarer than they once were. Many outstanding facilities exist that offer frail elderly people the medical and nursing care they need and treat their residents with dignity. But a nurs-

ing home is an institution, governed by regulations, both exter-
nally imposed (by state and federal agencies) and internally
imposed (by administrators seeking to run an efficient operation). The result is that nursing homes are seldom flexible: residents have to get up at specified times, bathe on prescribed days,
eat at predetermined hours. Privacy is a scarce commodity: the
majority of rooms are doubles. Residents usually share a bathroom. Doors are often left ajar so that staff can check on a resident's well-being as they walk down the halls. Even bathroom
doors are frequently left open to ensure the user's safety. Progressive institutions try to accommodate their residents' preferences
rather than force everyone into a single mold. But there are limits
to what even the most open-minded nursing home can achieve
with limited staff and a fixed physical plant.[4]

For Ben Frank, a very private man who sometimes liked to
watch the late-late show on television and sleep until ten A.M.,
moving into a nursing home would have been tremendously
restrictive. He knew he would be miserable if he lost his independence and his privacy, and he was frightened that that was
exactly what would happen to him. His son lived in a small apartment in Greenwich Village with his wife and daughter. Susan
lived in Boston, where he would be totally lost. Both of his children worked long hours and would not be able to take care of
him, even if they had the space. Moreover, he didn't want to burden them with the responsibility of looking after him. When
Carmela entered his life, he was as close to ecstatic as his supreme
reserve allowed him to be.

Not only was Ben far more relaxed once Carmela was in the
picture, but his children were calmer also. The nervous edge was
gone from Susan's voice. She wanted so badly to be a good
daughter, but had sometimes felt that whatever she did was not
enough. Her father didn't make her feel guilty—he appreciated

all her efforts on his behalf and thought she spent too many weekends traveling to see him. Her own conscience tormented her. When Susan chose to go away for a weekend with friends, only to return to a message from her brother on her answering machine that her father was back in the hospital, she felt as though his illness were her fault. Rationally, she knew that he would have fallen and developed a flare of his congestive heart failure whether she had been home or on vacation or, for that matter, even if she had been cooped up in his stuffy Bronx apartment. Nonetheless, the knowledge that she had been having a good time while he was suffering made her feel guilty. Hiring Carmela gave Susan peace of mind. Occasionally, she felt she ought to move to New York and take over her father's care. Most of the time she realized that would be a professional mistake. It would be a personal mistake as well—Carmela was far better at personal care than Susan was.

Perhaps it was no coincidence that Ben Frank became ill and was hospitalized again at just about the time he was beginnning to run out of the funds he needed to pay Carmela. When Susan told me about each new problem he developed in the hospital, she would always be optimistic that he would recover and be able to return home, where Carmela would resume her role as caregiver. The conviction that Carmela would be there for him helped sustain Susan through the cascade of catastrophes that comprised his final, two-month hospital stay.

Catherine Endicott

Catherine had chosen the apartment in Brookline for its location. It was the right size and was situated in an elevator building. Its major draw was that it was walking distance from a grocery store, a drugstore, and a library. Catherine's plan had been to do her own shopping and to volunteer at the library (and, incidentally, to check out books and attend some adult education programs)— and of course she needed a drugstore to maintain her supply of cardiac medications. The strategy was perfect—except that Catherine Endicott no longer had the strength to be self-sufficient.

After her hospitalization for angina and her successful angioplasty, her daughters were optimistic that she would be able to resume the simple existence she had carved out for herself. Surely a one-bedroom apartment was not too much to handle. Surely if Catherine concentrated exclusively on herself, she could manage.

The problem was that somewhere along the line—perhaps well before she entered the hospital and a new heart attack was "ruled out"—she had undoubtedly suffered further heart damage. One or two of her more prolonged episodes of chest pain, the ones that had lasted fifteen or twenty minutes, must have choked off just enough heart tissue to impair the heart's pumping action further. Now, even though Catherine had no more pain, she had hardly enough energy to prepare a meal for herself. She began eating a bowl of cereal for breakfast and heating up a can of soup for dinner. She skipped lunch entirely, occasionally treating herself to a cup of tea and a biscuit. Once an impeccable housekeeper, she gave up vacuuming and let a layer of grime accumulate on the bathtub. She did dust and she kept the apartment neat: that much she could do without expending a great deal of energy. She knew she was failing at living alone, so she tried to keep her daughters away. She did not want them to see the truth.

Jennifer made a surprise visit on Mother's Day and was appalled. Unwashed dishes were piled in the sink. The bed was unmade. The bathroom was visibly dirty. The refrigerator was empty except for half a quart of milk, a stick of margarine, and a few apples. When Jennifer asked if her mother had eaten anything that day—it was nearly four o'clock—Catherine broke down and cried.

Her two daughters took over the household management.

Within a matter of days they had hired a housekeeper to come in twice a week to clean, shop, and prepare a few dinners to be stored away for the next few days. They arranged for Meals-On-Wheels to deliver a hot meal five days a week. Jennifer and Andrea split the weekends, taking their mother to their own homes for a change of scene and a few home-cooked meals. Catherine no longer went hungry—she had lost ten pounds in two months—but she was starved for company. For the five days she was in the apartment by herself, her only companion was the housekeeper, a pleasant woman from Haiti whose English was marginal. Her daughters called daily, and the friends she had who still lived in the vicinity telephoned periodically. Everyone was busy tending to their medical problems or those of their spouses. Some of her friends had moved to Florida. A few had died. Catherine Endicott, a sociable woman who thrived on human contact, who had made a career of altruism, was lonely.

Her loneliness gradually turned into fearfulness. She left the radio on all night because she could not bear the quiet, but woke up in the middle of the night, frightened by the clanking of the radiator. She heard sounds in the hallway and was convinced her apartment was being broken into.

One night she awakened at five A.M., went to the bathroom, and felt short of breath. She returned to bed but refused to close her eyes, convinced she would never wake up again. She took her pulse. She made a wager: *If I'm still alive in five minutes, I'll make it to morning.* Catherine tried to remember the special breathing techniques her daughters had learned in childbirth classes—pant, pant, pant, pant, breathe. She found a focal point and tried to concentrate on it. She toyed with the idea of telephoning her daughters, but decided not to disturb them. It was still only five-thirty A.M. She tried to read but found she was mindlessly decoding the letters. She "read" three pages and realized she had no idea what she had read. In the distance, Catherine heard a siren. *Probably a fire,* she thought. The alarm gave her an idea. She rejected it first as too radical. But her reflexes took over and she could not stop herself. She picked up the receiver and dialed 911.

Within minutes, an ambulance pulled up in front of Catherine Endicott's apartment building. She scarcely noticed its arrival, since the driver had not used his siren—there was hardly any traffic at this hour. She heard the vigorous ringing of her doorbell, somehow managed to reach the buzzer to let the paramedics in, and the next thing she knew, two uniformed, reassuringly competent emergency medical technicians (EMTs) were in her living room.

"Chest pain?" one of them asked her by way of introduction.

Catherine shook her head. "Breathing trouble."

"Ever had congestive heart failure?" Catherine shook her head. "Ever had a heart attack?"

Catherine nodded. "I had angioplasty a couple of months ago." That seemed to seal the paramedics' decision. With a strong cardiac history and recent heart problems, they were not about to take any chances.

The second paramedic took Catherine's pulse and blood pressure, measured her respiratory rate, and briefly listened to her lungs. "Sounds pretty clear to me."

"Her respiratory rate is thirty-six, though," the first EMT observed. "Let's take her in." They lifted Catherine onto a stretcher, gave her oxygen through plastic tubing, and carried her out to the ambulance.

Catherine did not look particularly sick to the young doctors who greeted her in the emergency room. After a brief consultation with the attending physician, the more senior doctor supervising them, they decided the prudent course was to admit Catherine to the holding unit, an extension of the emergency room for patients who needed a few hours of observation. Her electrocardiogram was repeated several times, she had multiple blood tests, and she had a chest X ray.

After she had been in the holding unit for two hours, Andrea stormed in. She was angry at her mother for not having called her, she was angry at the emergency room doctors for not having simply admitted her mother to a regular hospital bed, and she was annoyed that they had not contacted her cardiologist.

The attending physician tried to calm her down. "Of course I'll call Dr. Fields to let him know your mother is here. But her electrocardiogram shows no changes, and her chest X ray is just fine. As a matter of fact, she felt much better as soon as she rolled through the door. I think what we have here is a case of nerves," he concluded.

Andrea was not satisfied until Dr. Fields himself delivered the same message. "She's fine. Take her home."

Andrea drove Catherine to her apartment and heated up lunch for the two of them in the microwave.

"You need to have more frequent checkups, Mom."

"I'm fine. You heard what the doctors said."

"But you haven't had an appointment in six weeks. Anything could happen in that time."

"Well, it didn't. And if it had, I doubt an extra visit would have made the difference."

"Mom, you're not taking care of yourself."

This provoked Catherine. "I don't do anything *but* take care of myself. I take my pills. I fix my meals. I don't do anything to strain myself." Andrea looked as though she was going to continue the argument, but her mother stopped her. "Enough. I'm going to bed." It had been a long day.

Jennifer had the idea of requesting that a visiting nurse come out to see Catherine once a week. She also asked for a physical therapist, since her mother was profoundly deconditioned after two months of restricting her activities to walking from the bed-room to the living room. She scheduled a follow-up visit with Dr. Fields. "I think everything will be okay now," Jennifer con-fided to her sister on the telephone. "She's got a visiting nurse and a physical therapist, a homemaker, and the Meals-On-Wheels. And us. I predict that within a month she'll be on her feet again."

Jennifer was mistaken. Before the month was up, Catherine again awoke in a panic during the night. She was sweating, her heart felt as though it were going to leap out of her chest, and she couldn't breathe. When it was all over, she had no recollection of calling the ambulance. The visit was a replay of her earlier one—more cardiograms, X rays, and blood tests. She got the same reas-surances that her heart was fine. This time she was sent home with a prescription for tranquilizers.

Andrea telephoned Dr. Fields. "Don't you think my mother should have another catheterization? How do you know that her arteries aren't blocked off again?"

Patiently, he explained that re-stenosis did occur and that, yes, Andrea was right that the most dangerous period was the first six months after angioplasty. But Catherine had had no chest pain, and all her tests had been strikingly normal. "Maybe you should take her to a psychiatrist."

Andrea was incensed. Her mother, who had retained her equa-nimity for the last seventy-seven years, did not need a psychia-trist. Why should she be anxious now, when she had no worries, no responsibilities, if she hadn't been anxious when she had to support her family and care for an ailing husband?

"Maybe she's afraid of dying," Jennifer suggested to her sister.

Andrea thought about that for a while. "Maybe she shouldn't live alone."

"I don't have enough room for her."

"I have the space, but I'm never around. She needs people around her."

A week later, Jennifer and Andrea presented their mother with a proposal. "We think you should move," Jennifer began.

"We found the perfect place for you. It's assisted living," Andrea continued.

"I don't need to move," Catherine countered.

"Just listen before you say no!" Jennifer insisted. "It's not a nursing home," she assured her mother. "You'd have your own apartment, just like here. But you'd eat in the dining room with everyone else—I think they have about one hundred apartments—three meals a day. They have housekeeping every week."

"That I already have," Catherine chimed in.

"And activities on site."

"Like what? Cards, I bet. And bingo. I'm not interested in cards and bingo."

"I brought along a schedule," Jennifer said, whipping it out of her pocket. "Look. Chamber music on Monday. A lawyer talking about long-term care insurance the next day. Waterpainting. Needlework. It sounds pretty good to me."

Catherine had no comment, so Jennifer continued. "They have movies every night. And a van to take people to appointments or out shopping. Andrea and I visited. It's a very attractive place." Catherine was not convinced that another move was either necessary or desirable, but she agreed to take a look.

"Everyone here is so old," was her only comment after seeing the facility. "They all look sick, with their walkers." And then, when her daughters' silence clearly indicated that they thought she would fit right in, she added, "It must be terribly expensive."

"It's not cheap," Andrea conceded. "They want three thousand dollars a month."

"Three thousand dollars a month?"

"Remember, that includes *everything*. That's not just rent. That's three meals a day—served in a dining room by waitresses. And heat and electricity and housekeeping. You won't have to pay anything else except your Medicare premiums."

"And clothes. And going to the beauty parlor."

"Well, of course there will be some extras. But it's more like staying in a hotel than on your own in an apartment."

"I have to think about it," Catherine told her children. "I need a little time."

What decided Catherine was not her daughters' persuasive arguments, nor the case made by the marketing representative at the assisted-living facility. What caused Catherine to make up her mind to move was Mary Shaughnessy.

Mary Shaughnessy, her husband, and their four children had rented the first floor of the triple-decker adjacent to the Endicotts' family house. It was only a two-bedroom apartment with a single bathroom, but for the Shaughnessy family it was a move up. Jim had grown up in the projects and was the first in his family to graduate from high school. Mary had worked as a house-cleaner until the twins came along. The twins were followed by two more children in three years. Jim had a decent job as a car mechanic, but he struggled to support his family. He did odd jobs as a handyman in the evenings to supplement his day job.

Over the next two decades, Catherine witnessed Mary's life unravel. The Shaughnessys did well for themselves until the twins started high school. Jim junior was recruited into the one gang that had penetrated the local high school. At sixteen he was smoking and taking drugs. At seventeen he dropped out of school. At eighteen he was in jail for dealing drugs. Jim's twin sister, Anne, became pregnant as a junior in high school and dropped out. For a time she lived at home with her parents, her siblings, and her baby. Then Jim junior was arrested, and she decided to move in with her boyfriend. He beat her up so badly that she feared for her life. She took her baby, moved out of the state, and never saw her parents again.

The two younger children, Kathleen and Kevin, were good students, and their parents were optimistic that they would be successful. Mary often confided to her neighbor, Catherine Endicott, that—God forgive her—she had given up on the twins, but she still had high hopes for her remaining children. Then Kevin was diagnosed with leukemia. Twenty years later, Catherine remembered the agony in Mary's voice when she told her about the visit to the doctor for swollen lymph glands, the fever that wouldn't go away, the fatigue, and the weight loss. Their family doctor had taken a blood test and sent Kevin to a specialist. The hematologist removed a specimen of bone marrow. The next day, the family got the report. Mary kept the household running, more or less, while she transported Kevin to and from his numerous medical appointments. He was treated with chemotherapy and went into remission. Six months later he relapsed. Again he got chemotherapy. His blood counts fell to dangerously low levels, and he developed pneumonia. He was hospitalized and vigorously treated, but the pneumonia spread to his other lung. In five days, he was comatose. Two weeks later, he was dead: bald, emaciated, his skin blotchy, his legs swollen.

After she lost Kevin, Mary began chain-smoking. Her husband started drinking. Within a year, he lost his job. In two years, he was found to have cirrhosis. In three years, Jim senior was dead. At age thirty-eight, Mary Shaughnessy was a widow. Her older son was in jail, her younger son was dead. Her older daughter sent her a Christmas card each year. All she had left was her seventeen-year-old daughter, who was getting failing grades in school and thinking of quitting.

A few evenings each week, Mary would drop by to see Catherine Endicott. Catherine was fifteen years her senior—a bit old to be a big sister to her, and a bit young to be a mother to her. Catherine had had her own share of troubles, with her husband's stroke, but she was a wonderful listener. It steadied Mary's nerves to sit in Catherine's kitchen and drink a cup of tea. Catherine was probably the only person in the world, with the possible exception of Mary's parish priest, who had confidence in Mary's ability to pull through.

Mary did survive after her husband's death, working once again by cleaning the homes of the middle class that she had aspired to join. She moved out of the sunny four-room apartment into a noisy, dark one-bedroom apartment in a different part of town. She continued to smoke heavily and was diagnosed with emphysema by the time she was in her fifties. The years of scrubbing floors took their toll, and she developed severe osteoarthritis. When Mary turned sixty-two, she was forced to stop working and go on disability. She was well on the road to frailty.

Catherine had moved out of town a few years earlier, but the two women stayed in touch. They had never been close—their worlds, their interests, their personalities, were too different. Nonetheless, there was a bond between them, derived from their both being women with sick husbands, working to support their families in an era when working women were not the norm. The two women spoke occasionally and exchanged letters from time to time.

Catherine was still thinking about assisted living when a headline in the living section of the newspaper caught her eye: "SIXTY-FIVE-YEAR-OLD WIDOW DIES OF SMOKE INHALATION," it read, with the subtitle "City's Frail Elderly Suffer from Neglect." Even before reading the heart-wrenching story that followed, Catherine was convinced that it was about Mary Shaughnessy.

The article described a woman who lived alone in a small apartment. She had emphysema, arthritis, and diabetes. As often happens in diabetics, she developed a foot ulcer: an open, festering wound. Her physician prescribed antibiotics and special dressings. The woman could not take care of the ulcer on her own, so a visiting nurse came to apply the dressing each day. The foot hurt, making it hard to walk around and tend to routine housekeeping chores. The woman was on Medicaid and was eligible for a homemaker twice a week. She relied on the homemaker to do her shopping and to clean. She ate tea and toast for breakfast and a can of soup for lunch. Often she skipped dinner. Other than the visiting nurse and the homemaker, she saw no one. Unbearably lonely and in pain, her only solace was cigarettes. One evening, she dozed off while smoking. The apartment went up in flames, and the woman died of smoke inhalation. The woman's name was not released until two days later, when, after considerable difficulty, her children were traced. It was Mary Shaughnessy.

Mary's life had always seemed like a soap opera—one unmitigated disaster after another. Catherine was haunted by the image of Mary in pain, Mary short of breath, Mary with a foul-smelling sore on her foot. Worst of all, she kept thinking that Mary had lived alone, suffered alone, and died alone. That settled matters for her. Catherine decided she would prefer a more communal living arrangement to the anonymous building in which she lived.

Catherine Endicott agreed to move to assisted living. Her daughters would orchestrate the move, ensuring that all her possessions were transferred to the corresponding locations in the new apartment. The only substantive modification in her living quarters would be that she would have just the tiniest of kitchenettes. She was not expected to do any of her own cooking—the stove would merely allow her to boil water for tea, and the mini-refrigerator would enable her to store a few snacks. She would take meals in the dining room. The other major difference between the two buildings was in the extensiveness of the communal facilities. In her new home, Catherine would have privacy but never be truly alone.

Jennifer and Andrea were more anxious about the move than their mother was. Once Catherine had made her decision, she had no second thoughts. That was the way Catherine was—she thought long and hard about things, but did not replay her deliberations once she reached a conclusion. Her acquaintances sometimes said she was a great rationalizer, always finding everything for the best. Her close friends knew that was not true; she was simply a pragmatist. She understood that there were certain things she couldn't change and she didn't pretend she could. Catherine did not play "what if" games; she took reality as her point of departure, and tried to optimize her moves.

Perhaps her daughters were especially anxious about the move because they felt responsible. They sensed that if anything went wrong, Catherine would have to move in with one of them. Perhaps they were a little sad because they realized this would be the last stop for their mother on her life's journey. Or maybe they were just frazzled because they had made the arrangements with the moving company and the telephone company and the post office and were worried that something would go wrong.

Remarkably, everything fell into place. The movers showed up more or less on time and the phone company managed to disconnect the old phone line and activate the new one without any significant disruption of service. The new apartment was ready, as promised: the rugs had been shampooed and the walls repainted. Unpacking did not take long, since by now Catherine was traveling quite light. She had thrown out or given away most of her material possessions on the occasion of the first move. This move went so smoothly that Catherine managed to shower and change in time to have dinner in the main dining room.

To her astonishment, she met an old neighbor on her first evening in the assisted-living complex. She had not seen Elizabeth Garber for thirty years, but they recognized each other instantly. Beth's history was very similar to Catherine's—childhood in the same town, a move upon getting married, but then a return to the family's house. Beth and her husband and son had moved to the same town where Catherine had lived most recently. They had used the same library and convenience store, though they had never run into each other. Beth had just lost her husband and, rather than remaining in her seven-room house by herself, had opted for assisted living.

The two widows ate dinner together and reminisced. Actually, Beth did most of the talking and Catherine most of the listening. Catherine had the impression that even when she said something, Beth was too self-absorbed to pay much attention. Nonetheless, it was comforting to have a compatriot in what felt like a new land.

After dinner, Catherine was too tired to go to the nightly movie, although Beth urged her to come along. "It's Ginger Rogers. Every Wednesday they have old movies. *Singin' in the Rain* was last week. Don't you love that film? It's a big screen in what they call the parlor. No noisy children and no popcorn. Don't you find the smell of popcorn dreadful?" Catherine noticed that all of Beth's questions were rhetorical, or at least she never allowed enough time for an answer.

"Another time. Next Wednesday. I'm tired."

Beth shook her head. "Lots of the old ladies here, they sleep their lives away. Turn in for the night by eight o'clock." It was seven-thirty. "Don't they realize they don't have much time left? They should squander it on sleep?" She clucked. "I'm eighty years old. Eighty last April. How much longer can I have? My dear husband, may he rest in peace, was eighty-four when he died. For a whole year, he was sick and I nursed him. It wasn't easy—"

"I took care of my husband for seventeen years," Catherine interrupted. She wasn't usually fond of one-upmanship, but Beth's sanctimonious boasting was too irritating for her to ignore. "My philosophy is work hard during the day and get a good night's sleep. Good night, Beth." Catherine made her way to her new apartment slowly, leaning heavily on her cane. She noticed that quite a number of the tenants used walkers, and wondered fleetingly whether she would be better off with more support. She had slowed down tremendously since the angioplasty. Her doctor had muttered something about "senile gait disorder," in which the nerves controlling the fluid, coordinated movements necessary for walking were disordered. She had recently developed claudication—she got cramps in her legs when she walked, a kind of angina of the leg muscles. It wasn't just her walking that had slowed down. After Catherine unlocked the front door, she spent an hour getting ready for bed. Everything took longer than it had previously—undressing, washing up—and of course there were all the new additions to her routine, like removing her dentures and taking her evening medications.

Catherine wondered whether she would wake up in a sweat at five A.M. and, if so, what she would do. Before she finished speculating, she was in a deep, untroubled sleep.

Catherine discovered that she knew several tenants in the assisted-living complex, not just the garrulous Beth. Like her, they had spent their lives near the town where she grew up, though most had moved to one or another nearby suburb. Their sons and daughters had become professionals—teachers and bankers, doctors and lawyers. Their mothers were very proud of them, but their success meant they were too busy to be able to take care of a frail, aging parent. They had all remained at home until some crisis supervened: most commonly the loss of a spouse (as with Beth); or, alternatively, illness; or sometimes overweening anxiety (as with Catherine). They were all grateful for assisted living.

Beth was endlessly critical of the complex where she lived. "The management is terrible," she explained to Catherine on her first full day. "They've been through three directors in six months. Not a good sign." Catherine just listened. "The waiters and waitresses are all very young, very inexperienced. I think they pay them minimum wage. You can get away with that in a restaurant, where the staff gets tips every night. But here—this is where we live! If I had the same waitress all year, I would give her a little something at Christmas. But they come and go so fast, I don't even have time to learn their names. First it was Molly, I think. She left after a few weeks to get a real waitressing job, once she could say she had experience. Then came Laura—no, I think it was Ellen, but it might have been Laura." Catherine dozed off and Beth, after continuing her monologue a little longer, decided to search for a more attentive audience.

In truth, Beth's critique was on target. The facility was poorly run, and whenever someone competent was hired—a creative activities leader, for example—she didn't last long. The housekeepers were a sullen lot. They were ill-equipped to deal with the tenants, some of whom were demanding, and some of whom were cognitively impaired. Tenants were excluded if they had advanced dementia, but many were in the early stages of

Alzheimer's disease. They had to be able to get to the dining room three times a day, they had to be socially appropriate, and they could not wander aimlessly, at risk of getting lost. They could not live in the assisted-living facility if they had major physical disabilities. They received only forty minutes a day of personal assistance, which amounted to little more than help showering and dressing. Residents who needed more help than the system was designed to provide, or who needed little bits of assistance throughout the day, were asked to leave.

The exclusionary policy was the topic of much of the residents' dinnertime conversation. On the one hand, those who had their wits about them were less than kind to those residents who asked the same questions repeatedly, whose table manners were atrocious, or who came to meals with mismatched socks and their shirts inside out. On the other hand, they were terrified that they would be asked to leave if they forgot their keys or missed a meal or showed any other signs of a failing memory.

"That Sylvia Truman doesn't belong here," Beth asserted one evening over coffee. "She smells."

Catherine, who scarcely knew who Sylvia Truman was, rushed to her defense as a matter of principle. "Maybe she has a bladder problem."

"Obviously she has a bladder problem!"

"Well, lots of women have bladder trouble after they've had several babies." This was a sore point for Beth, who had had only one child and had given birth by Cesarean section. "I only had two and I was stretched out of shape pretty badly," Catherine continued. "Also, my girls were small. My friends who had three, including a couple of boys, they all have a dropped bladder."

Beth changed the subject. "Did you hear they ran out of chicken last night? Some people had to have beans and hot dogs!" Catherine was less interested in defending the management, so

she let Beth continue her attack. Others were more forgiving of
the facility's administration.

"It's not so easy figuring out how much to get for a hundred
people."

"At a restaurant they figure it out."

"Restaurants run out, too, sometimes. Also, they have lots of
choices, so odds are there won't be a run on any one thing. Here
there are only two choices for the entrée. If three-quarters of the
residents want the same thing, they've got a problem."

"So they should have more than two main courses to choose
from. If they had three, I bet they wouldn't run out."

It was impossible to win an argument against Beth. But all four
ladies who had grown up together agreed—at some level, even Beth
agreed—that assisted living was working out very well for them.
Other people didn't belong there. *Other* people found the activities
either too tedious or too sophisticated. The four of them felt more
relaxed, more secure, and more contented than they had in a long
time. Beth called her son only once a day to complain instead of
three times a day, as she had previously. The other two women, both
of whom had been treated for depression after their husbands died,
no longer saw their psychiatrists and were off antidepressant medication. Catherine never again dialed 911 or summoned her daughters to take her to the emergency room. All of them enjoyed each
other's company and, when they had had enough of each other,
appreciated the opportunity to retreat to the privacy of their own
apartments.

Jack Simon

For all their bravado, Jack's children had never been convinced
that their father would be safe at home after his stroke. The crisis

that they had been sure would come eventually arrived three months after his cataract surgery. It was a modest catastrophe, as catastrophes go, and it did not involve Jack directly; it centered on his wife. Margaret fell and broke her wrist. She had a Colles' fracture, one of the most common types of fracture in older women. Women with osteoporosis were at especially high risk for a Colles' fracture, and older white women with a narrow build were at high risk of osteoporosis. Margaret Simon was seventy-eight, white, and petite. She took calcium pills faithfully every day, which may have contributed to her having reached seventy-eight without prior fractures.[5]

The treatment involved a cast, initially extending above the elbow. Margaret was right-handed, and with her arm in a cast, she had difficulty dressing herself. She could not drive to do the shopping. She could not cook or clean. She certainly could not help Jack get washed or dressed.

The three empty upstairs bedrooms came in handy, as did a small reserve fund in the bank. Margaret hired twenty-four-hour live-in help to take care of the two of them. Fortunately, virtually no assistance proved necessary at night, which made the job quite tolerable for the young Irish woman they hired. She had original-ly come to the United States as an au pair, but found the two-year-old twins in her care insufferable and exhausting. Mr. and Mrs. Simon, by contrast, who tried to do everything for them-selves and called upon her only when they were stymied by their respective handicaps, were a delight. Orla was relieved to find herself in a less demanding job, but after a few weeks she began to get restless. She wanted to travel, to explore America, not just to learn what it was like to lead a suburban existence. She did not want to leave Margaret and Jack in the lurch, so she agreed to stay until Margaret's cast came off.

The day after the cast was removed, Orla left for New Orleans.

She had heard about the French Quarter and the Mardi Gras and was itching to go. Promising to write—she did send one postcard—Orla took off on her adventure.

"I've made a decision," Jack told Margaret, somewhat ominously, one night as they sat down to dinner. "I think we should move."

"Why? You don't think I can cope without Orla?"

"I think it will be rough. We could find another Orla, but I think the house is just too big for us."

"Where would you want to move to?"

"I've gotten some literature on continuing-care retirement communities. There's a fairly new one not far from here. We'd have our own apartment, two meals a day in the dining room, plenty to do on the premises, but also our privacy."

"You mean live in a segregated apartment building, with a bunch of old people?"

"We're old people, Peggy." Jack reached for his wife's hand. "It seems to me we mainly socialize with people our age anyway. The advantage of a place like Park Village is that there's a lot of help available—if we need it. There's even a nursing home on the premises for temporary problems."

"Those places always have such bucolic names: Park or Green or Meadow. That's because they're places you go to when you've been put out to pasture."

"Margaret, how about if we visit? What's there to lose?"

Peggy did not like the idea, but she reluctantly visited two continuing-care retirement communities with Jack in tow—one in a neighboring town, the other a half hour's drive. They also visited an assisted-living complex in the neighborhood, a facility intended for more disabled individuals. The assisted-living complex and the continuing-care retirement communities (CCRC) operated on different financial bases. In assisted living, you were assessed a monthly fee. It was a steep fee, amounting to $4,000 for a unit for two people, which included half an hour per day of personal care for each of them, plus a full meal plan. The apartment had two bedrooms, a small living room, and a tiny kitchenette adequate for preparing snacks but not full meals. The continuing-care retirement communities, by contrast, featured larger, more luxurious apartments and extensive grounds. Each apartment came with a parking space, since the residents were clearly expected to be independent and active. In addition to the hefty one-time purchase fee of $250,000 (which was refundable on moving out), there was a monthly service charge. For a larger service charge, residents could also obtain personal-care services, making the arrangements equivalent to assisted living. A skilled nursing home was on site as a backup in the event a resident developed an acute illness or for rehabilitation after a hip fracture or stroke.

The sales representative at the first CCRC conveyed the impression that he had previously worked as a used-car salesman. He wheedled, exaggerated, and generally came across as entirely untrustworthy. The facility itself was very attractive, but Margaret was skeptical. She wondered how sound a financial footing the institution had. Suppose the place went bankrupt. The residents would not get their "deposit" back if they moved out, nor would their children inherit the money when they died. That nice security blanket—the on-site nursing home—would not do you any good if it folded. She was dubious about the vaunted comprehensive nursing and medical care. Residents were expected to get their doctoring from the facility's affiliated physician group, much as though they were joining a health-maintenance organization. Were the doctors any good? Were they specialists in geriatrics? Were they internists without any particular interest in the elderly who merely wanted to pad their rolls?

At the assisted-living facility, Jack and Peggy were given a tour by a young, inexperienced woman who was honest about how little she knew. She readily admitted her ignorance when asked probing questions: No, she did not know what fraction of the residents had dementia. She had no idea what the staff-turnover rate was. She knew the fees had gone up 2 percent for the current year, but did not know the extent of previous increases. Peggy was unimpressed. Jack argued that if they were seriously interested, surely they could meet with someone who could answer their questions. They decided, however, that they were not interested: it was a facility overwhelmingly devoted to individuals who did not have a spouse and who, in general, were considerably more impaired than Jack was.

Park Village, the second CCRC, was more promising. They met with the director, not a salesperson on commission or a college student working as a tour guide. The director was knowledgeable, sophisticated, and compassionate. He understood that the decision to sell one's house and enter a retirement village was emotionally traumatic. It involved moving—itself a major upheaval. More important, it was a highly symbolic move, representing the beginning of the last chapter of life. The CCRC was typically the last stop before the cemetery, and while many retired elderly people could look forward to years of fulfillment, they knew their days were numbered. They would, moreover, be living exclusively with their peers and would constantly see what might be in store for them: illness, progressive disability, and death.

"It's so *final*," Peggy explained to her daughter, Ginny. "Once you've sold your house and bought into this, there's no turning back."

"You could change your mind," Ginny disagreed. "You couldn't move back to your old house, but, then again, you and Dad have already agreed the house is too big and not designed for your needs. And it's not as though you have so many friends in the neighborhood anymore. Len Wolf died and his wife moved in with their daughter. The Martins moved to Florida. The Jacksons moved away to be near their children. I can't think of anyone you're really close to who is still around."

"But I love this house. This is where you grew up. Doesn't it mean anything to you?" Peggy spoke accusingly.

"It does mean a lot to me. But it's more important to see you and Dad in a safe, comfortable environment."

Peggy found a succession of excuses for not taking the plunge: first it was that the house needed some cosmetic work before she could even think of putting it on the market; then it was that everyone said winter was a terrible time to put a house up for sale; then it was that she could not concentrate on anything until after income tax day. On April 16, Jack had a surprise waiting for Peggy when she returned from her weekly supermarket trip: a realtor had come to assess their house. There were only a handful of suitable apartments still available at Park Village. Jack had assembled all the papers. In an orgy of signatures, the Simons agreed to sell the home they had lived in for forty-five years and move to a CCRC. Their son Mark was in town, so they all went out to dinner to celebrate, Mark helping with transportation.

For sentimental reasons, they ate at a nearby Italian restaurant to which Jack and Margaret had been loyal during its many incarnations. Originally a French bistro, it had been reborn as an Indian restaurant (too spicy for local tastes), and then as an Irish pub (too rowdy for the neighborhood). The current owner had been in business for two years and did not know the Simon family since they had not dined out very often during his tenure.

They enjoyed the veal scallopini and the eggplant parmigiana and treated themselves to wine since Mark was driving. They found it simultaneously comforting to be in a familiar environment and disturbing that none of the waiters knew them. They were strangers in their own land. It was a fitting transition to their new home.

The house was sold remarkably quickly. "Flexible floor plan," the realtor proclaimed in her ad, in recognition of the fact that Jack's bedroom was downstairs. "In-law possibility," she added, since there was now a full bathroom on the first floor. A couple with two small children made an offer—they wanted the downstairs bedroom for a nanny and they liked the yard and the neighborhood. Lots of young families had moved into the area as houses were vacated by Jack and Peggy's generation. The new prospective owners wanted to move over the summer, so as to be ensconced by the beginning of the school year. Before Labor Day, the Simons were in their new home.

If Peggy was ambivalent beforehand, she was no more convinced that they had made the right choice after the fact. The apartment, she admitted, was beautiful. They had kept some of their furniture but bought a few new pieces, including an armchair that Jack could get out of, unlike their old armchairs, which were so soft and low to the ground that once Jack was seated he could not get up by himself. The floors were freshly carpeted with Berber rugs, nothing so plush that Jack's walker—which he used for short distances—would get stuck. The walls were covered with cheery new wallpaper boasting trees and flowers, in keeping with the park motif. The rooms were exceptionally bright, as the architect had included enough skylights and recessed lights to be sure the apartment was well illuminated by day and by night.

Their neighbors, Peggy reluctantly conceded, were lovely people. Well educated and engaged in numerous volunteer projects, they were warm and gracious toward the new arrivals. Peggy and Eleanor quickly became friends, as did Jack and Sidney. They made it a habit to sit together in the communal dining room at least once a week. Sidney insisted that Jack join him in the CCRC's exercise program. Eleanor even persuaded Peggy to join her on one of her outings, which meant convincing her that the monthly book club was worth attending and that she could safely leave Jack by himself.

Not everyone in the "Village" was to their liking. "It's a little like going to college and being thrust into a dormitory with all sorts of people," Peggy explained to her son Stuart when he came to visit. "Some of them you don't particularly care for. Of course we have a lot more privacy than in a dormitory. Even at meal-times, we eat together but we're in a dining room, not a cafeteria. We don't have to mingle with anyone we'd rather not be with. It is sort of a gossipy place," Peggy mused. "Everyone seems to know what everyone else is doing. Some of the residents are real busy-bodies. And the staff are nosy, too. They're apparently worried about the Village's image, and want to weed out people with any signs of Alzheimer's disease. At first they weren't too pleased about Dad, with his walker and his wheelchair. I think they were reluctant to accept us."

Stuart laughed. "That was a good thing. It was only when they suggested that you two were too feeble for them that you concluded everyone else at Park Village must be in pretty good shape, good enough to satisfy you."

Peggy reluctantly acknowledged that there was some truth to what Stuart said. Only when they nearly failed the admissions screen did Peggy become adamant that they be accepted. "I had to prove to them that Dad's brains and sense of humor made up for his trouble walking. I also mumbled something about the Americans with Disabilities Act and getting a lawyer. They backed down after that."

Stuart beamed at his mother. His father was smart, Stuart thought, but his mother was the really sharp one in the family.

She had only graduated from high school, married early, and devoted most of her energy as a young woman to raising her three children. If she had been born in another time and another place, Stuart believed, she would have pursued a professional career. She could have done anything she set her mind to—medicine, law, academia. What she had in fact set her mind to was her family, and she had done a very good job with them.

The Village recruited a series of dynamic speakers to present lectures followed by what was usually an animated discussion. The residents debated political issues like term limits, they heard about living wills, and they argued about a proposal to build a halfway house in their neighborhood. They listened attentively and spoke out passionately, whether the issue appealed to their self-interest or not. Jack and Peggy, whose only stimulation for more than a year had been newspapers, radio programs, and the Sturm und Drang of their own medical dilemmas, blossomed.

Jack had often felt inadequate among highly educated people. He had wanted desperately to be a podiatrist, but just when he finished high school, the Depression hit and he had to work to support his parents. He managed to take a few business courses in night school, which helped as he worked himself up from factory worker to supervisor to salesman. Jack had enjoyed mingling with the company's executives and, better yet, with his counterparts at other companies whom he met on his travels. They took him out when he came to town, entertained him, and shared some of their worldliness. At Park Village, Jack was uninhibited. He was a man of experience; he had done reasonably well economically. He could hold his own at any dinner table.

After considerable trial and error, Peggy found a suitable activity for herself, apart from tending to Jack. She became involved in the local literacy campaign, tutoring reading. Her particular forte, she discovered, was working with adults who had never learned to read. School-age children were too impatient with her, but adults liked her, finding the typical instructor intimidating. Peggy was a nonjudgmental, grandmotherly figure who made her students feel appreciated whether or not they succeeded in reading. Once the fear of failure dissipated, they took greater risks and achieved correspondingly more than students working with other teachers. Peggy was especially proud of Jared Symes, a twenty-nine-year-old man who was tall and strong and walked with a swagger. Underneath his cocky exterior, he felt insecure and incompetent. In his community, he tried to hide the fact that he had never learned to read. In his experience, there were two types of people: those who respected him because he was tough, and those who looked down on him because he was illiterate. Peggy was a different species. She had no interest in his street skills, but seemed to like him despite his inability to read.

Jared had missed a great deal of school in the elementary years. Both his parents were alcoholics. His father beat his mother when he was drunk, and squandered what little money he earned on reconciliation gifts when he was sober. Whether Jared went to school depended on whether his parents were too hung over to take him. When he was in second grade, his father left and he never saw him again. What followed was a series of moves from one roach-infested apartment to another. Each time they moved, he had to change schools, and sometimes his mother was too tired or disorganized or depressed to bother enrolling him in the neighborhood school. He ended up missing six months of third grade altogether. By the time he was nine years old, his mother had taken up with a new man. The relationship lasted three years, during which time Jared attended school continuously. He did not know how to read, but after each year he was promoted to the next grade. He sat in class, increasingly bored and bewildered, dreaming of becoming a basketball star.

Peggy was furious at the public schools that had failed Jared so miserably. She was appalled that he had moved through the system without anyone noticing or caring about how little he had learned. She was pained that he had spent so many hours of his childhood hopelessly bored. She was touched that despite his years of being lost, he wanted someone to find him and teach him how to read.

The first month they worked together, Jared made no discernible progress in reading, though he made extensive invisible progress, like a plant growing roots before it develops shoots. He learned to trust Peggy, despite the fact that he had trusted few adults before. They made an odd couple: he was tall, young, and black; she was small, old, and white. What they had in common was that they were both sure that no stranger would find them the slightest bit interesting. They were both mistaken.

After four sessions together in the Park Village common room, there was a breakthrough. Peggy realized that the whole-language method of reading instruction, in which she had been coached by the leaders of the literacy project, was useless for Jared. The approach was predicated on the student's willingness to guess a word from context, based on knowing some of the letters. Jared refused to guess: his difficulty was precisely that he would not take risks, at least not in the literary domain. Peggy noticed that he knew the sound of every consonant in the alphabet; it was only the vowels that eluded him. She praised him profusely for his proficiency, pointing out that he was very comfortable with twenty-one out of twenty-six letters. They worked on vowels between breaks for tea and cookies. In another two weeks, Jared started to read.

Peggy's next project was to coach her protégé in applying for a job. She helped him, and a few of his marginally literate friends, to complete job applications. Jack helped as well, drawing on his experience coaching middle-aged executives. They set up the Simon and Simon Vocational Counseling Service. They had very few clients, most of whom were connected in some fashion to Jared Symes, but they found the work exhilarating. They credited Park Village with giving them a home from which to operate, and a secure environment that enabled Peggy to venture outside.

Leyla Keribar

After her recovery from hip-replacement surgery due to osteo-arthritis, Leyla Keribar did well for a period of close to a year. She seemed more accepting of her physical condition, and she stopped complaining quite so vociferously about the garden apartment in which she lived. Her Parkinson's disease remained stable, and she had no recurrence of depression. Just as Valerie was congratulating herself that her mother was doing well, she discovered that Leyla was becoming progressively more anxious. She worried whenever Valerie deviated in the slightest from her usual routine, even if she came home late from work.

"But Mom, I'm not a child anymore! Sometimes I get stuck in traffic. Sometimes I stop at the market to pick up fresh fruit on the way home. You don't need to worry about me." But Leyla worried, and Valerie began to make it a habit to call every day before she left work to report her plans.

Leyla worried about her grandson. She stayed up waiting for him when he went out on dates. Once she sat in the living room with the lights off, waiting. He walked in, flicked on the switch, and was taken aback to find her sitting primly in the armchair, her eyes wide open. He was irritated—what if he'd had his girlfriend with him? What if he had kissed his girlfriend in the dark and then noticed his grandmother, perched motionless like an

owl ready to swoop down on its prey? He told her sharply that
her behavior was scandalous. Even his parents trusted him and no
longer stayed up for him in the evening. From then on, she sat up
waiting in the garden apartment.

When her younger grandson left for college, Leyla's anxiety
escalated. "I'm supposed to suffer from empty nest syndrome,
not you!" Valerie said, anguished, to her mother. "And it's hard
for me. But having you worried all the time makes it doubly
hard."

"I can't help it," Leyla told her daughter. For a time, she had
her grandsons calling her twice a week and Valerie every day from
work. But she began to forget whether the boys had called her
yet. The system that was supposed to reassure her backfired, as
she was forever awaiting someone's call and did not derive satisfaction from the calls because she did not remember her conversations.

Reminders helped jog her memory. "Josh isn't going to call
this week, Mom. He went on a trip to Memphis to meet his girlfriend's parents." Leyla would acknowledge she'd been told that
before. "Alex spoke to you yesterday. Remember, he told you he
got an A on that paper he'd been so worried about?" Leyla
remembered that, too. Without the reminders, she became pan-
icky. She spent most of her day beside the telephone, anticipating
its ring.

"I move slowly, so I'm afraid I won't get there in time," she
explained.

"We all know to let it ring. The only people who hang up after
two or three rings are the solicitors you don't want to talk to anyway," Valerie commented. But Leyla was obsessed with the
importance of her proximity to the telephone. Valerie bought her
a cordless telephone, but she was too flustered to press the ON
button when it rang and often neglected to press the OFF button

after a conversation. She continued to spend most of her day in her apartment, next to the phone, waiting.

Perhaps because she was so close to the phone all the time, Leyla developed a new habit: at least once a day, she called her daughter at work in a frenzy. "I can't find my keys," she would report, although she didn't particularly need her keys since she wasn't planning to go anywhere. Or: "I heard on the radio there was a car accident on the interstate and I was convinced you'd been hurt," even though Valerie was seldom on the road at that time and almost never drove on the highway in question.

Valerie and George pondered at length the precipitant for Leyla's escalating anxiety. Valerie thought it was related to her younger son being out of the house—despite his extracurricular activities, he had often come home in the afternoon, so his grandmother could look forward to another person in the house. Even when they did not converse, Leyla had found his presence soothing. Since the high school was in walking distance of the house, he had sometimes come home for lunch and then gone back to school. They had eaten together in the kitchen—as a real treat, he would make a vegetable omelet for the two of them, or a grilled cheese sandwich. Leyla had lived for those lunches, when he would pour out his adolescent troubles to her far more freely than he would to his parents. Parents commented and criticized. Grandmothers, or at least this one, just listened, delighted to glimpse into the soul of the next generation. The lunches had been like a long-acting medication for Leyla, maintaining her sense of importance for as much as a week at a time. Now her grandson was in college five hundred miles away and she saw him an average of three times a year.

George thought the trigger was his mother-in-law's failing memory. Once a brilliant woman, she had lost her sharp edge. She was still clearly an intelligent woman, and Valerie at first had difficulty believing her mother's mind was weakening. Gradually, the signs became unmistakable. She would ask the same question three times in five minutes. She did not remember momentous news she had learned the previous day. She misplaced things. One day she set out in the middle of the night, walking in the pouring rain with no umbrella and no raincoat. When a policeman stopped her to ask where she was headed, she couldn't tell him. She knew her address, so he bundled her into his squad car and brought her home.

Valerie was mortified—alarmed that her mother might have hurt herself, and chagrined that she had apparently not provided adequate supervision. She felt like a mother whose two-year-old had run off on the beach and gotten lost. She concluded that Leyla could no longer be left alone. She required a companion twenty-four hours a day. Valerie considered hiring a live-in aide for her mother, but her house, for all its size, was not set up to accommodate a housekeeper. The companion could, Valerie supposed, live in the garden apartment with Leyla, sleeping in the living room, but that arrangement would afford no privacy for either of them. The companion could live in the garden apartment and Leyla could move into one of the boys' old bedrooms, which her mother would probably applaud since she had never adjusted to her "exile." That solution would destroy precisely what the garden apartment had been designed to achieve: it would ensure that the three of them would once again be on top of one another. The other flaw in the companion idea was that Leyla would remain socially isolated.

George arrived at the answer over dinner. "I think Leyla should go into a nursing home."

Valerie was stunned. "You're just tired of her. You want to get rid of her."

"Have I ever complained? Did I protest when your parents first moved in with us? Did I give you a hard time about moving just for them?"

Chastened, Valerie had to admit that he had always been extraordinarily accepting.

"But why do you think she needs a nursing home?"

"She has Parkinson's and has trouble walking. When she does walk, her joints bother her. She's eighty years old and she is consumed by anxiety. And now she's getting dementia." He had said it. He had said what had been on their minds for weeks.

"But George, I can't put her in a nursing home! I've always said I would take care of her. I can't abandon her."

"You wouldn't be abandoning her. We'll find a nice place where she gets good care. You'll visit her regularly. You'll probably enjoy being with her much more than you do now, because you won't have to take care of her, you'll just *be* with her."

Valerie started to cry. It simultaneously sounded so right and so terribly wrong. The subject was closed for the evening.

Two weeks later Valerie began making inquiries about nursing homes. She casually mentioned to her mother that she was looking around.

"I know where I want to go," Leyla told her directly.

"You what?" Valerie thought perhaps she had misunderstood.

"I used to volunteer at the Turkish Home for the Aged. Do you remember?"

Valerie did remember. Her mother helped the residents make baklava for special occasions.

"I think I would be comfortable there. It would be very familiar."

One of the potentially devastating consequences of moving into a nursing home is losing the ties to one's culture. It is hard enough to move into an institution—to give up one's own home and be forced to adapt to a life of regimentation. It is hard enough to be arbitrarily assigned a roommate in your eighties when, unlike in the college years, living with a stranger is scarcely an educational experience. It is difficult enough to accept one's frailty, for frailty, whether physical, mental, or both, is generally the reason for entering a nursing home. To have to eat food cooked with unfamiliar spices, or perhaps even forbidden by one's religious tradition, could make a difficult life intolerable. To live in a home where other people's holidays are celebrated but not your own is alienating and lonely.[6]

Valerie and Leyla went together to visit the Turkish Home. Seeing the place through the eyes of a prospective resident was, after all, very different from seeing it from the perspective of a volunteer. It was an old building, a little shabby. The wallpaper was torn in spots, the linoleum was worn. But it was clean, it was neat, and it boasted a few homey touches. There was a fireplace in the common room, a gathering spot for the residents. The fire was electric, but from a distance it looked real enough. There were plants in the dining room, much to the dismay of the wait staff, who felt they cluttered a room already filled with walkers and canes. Photographs of Istanbul and Ankara lined the hallways.

The highlight of their visit was not the tour of the facilities, nor was it the strong Turkish coffee the social worker gave them during her intake interview. The highlight of the trip—what sold Leyla on the place—was what they learned about the nursing staff.

"There is a nurse on duty all day?" she asked, incredulous. Their tour guide nodded. "At night, too?"

"There's a registered nurse on duty twenty-four hours a day, on each floor. The number of aides varies, depending on the shift. Days we have four aides for forty residents on the floor where you would live. Evenings we have two aides, and nights we have only one." *Days,* Valerie would soon learn, meant from seven A.M. to three P.M.; *evenings* spanned the period from three

P.M. to eleven P.M., and *nights* implied the eleven P.M. to seven A.M. shift.

Leyla pressed for further clarification. "So, if I need help I just call the nurse?"

"That's right. Though mainly it's the nursing assistant assigned to you who will help you out. She has nine other residents to take care of, so you might have to wait a little. But yes, staff is always here to attend to your needs." Until that point during the visit, Leyla had been passive, dutifully looking at whatever was pointed out to her as she was driven around the premises in a wheelchair. Now she became more animated.

"At night, too?" she persevered.

"At night, too," the social worker repeated.

Lately, Leyla had had increasing trouble being alone. It was no longer enough for her to know that her family was in the house with her: she had to see them. Whenever she heard her daughter or son-in-law in the house, she wanted their company. Valerie found herself rushing to her mother's side in response to a frantic yell, only to find that she did not know or could not remember what she wanted. A nursing home seemed like the perfect solution to Leyla's unquenchable thirst for companionship.

Once Leyla actually moved into the nursing home, she did not find it quite the utopia she had imagined. She continued telephoning Valerie at work. She even began telephoning George, which she had never done before. She left messages of desperation on his answering machine. Each time he felt compelled to call the nurses' station, just to make sure his mother-in-law was not in fact dying, or to double-check that the nursing aide hadn't really forgotten to get her dressed. Leyla once said she was "terribly sick"; he called and learned she had a cold. One day she claimed the staff was "neglecting her"; he found out that she was scheduled for a mid-morning shower, so the protracted dressing routine had been postponed until after bathing. The messages, however implausible, were always so sincere, so compelling, that they demanded a response.

Valerie and George were rational people, and they were compassionate toward the staff, though their primary focus, of course, remained Leyla. They apologized to the nurses for their frequent calls—and for Leyla's incessant demands. They took Leyla out to lunch every week, and they accompanied her to concerts and other entertainment provided by the nursing home. They brought fruit and candy for the staff. Gradually, they all adjusted to each other's idiosyncrasies.

Together, staff and family worked out a system to keep the telephone calls under control. Valerie called her mother every day at eleven A.M. The grandsons came up with a weekly calling schedule. Visits were similarly planned in advance. As Leyla became more forgetful, Valerie made a special calendar listing all the important daily events, and the staff checked off whenever calls came in.

A psychiatric consultant made suggestions regarding medication to take the edge off Leyla's anxiety. Choosing a drug was tricky: the neuroleptic medicines the psychiatrist initially favored aggravated her Parkinson's disease. Leyla could not even tolerate the newer variants that were touted as being less likely to cause rigidity. The psychiatrist next recommended a trial of an antidepressant, since Leyla had been depressed before, and depression frequently recurred. He thought her calling out might be an atypical manifestation of depression. Valerie pointed out that her mother had been on several different antidepressants at the time of her suicide gesture, none of which had agreed with her. This time she took Prozac, a medication with a different mechanism of action from older, traditional antidepressants. Mercifully, it didn't produce any side effects, but it also had no discernible beneficial effect. Antianxiety drugs such as Ativan (lorazepam) and Serax (oxazepam) made Leyla excessively sleepy, impaired her already tenuous balance, and, in the doses she could tolerate, had no effect whatsoever on her calling out. Finally, the psychiatrist hit upon Buspar (buspirone), an antianxiety medication with mild antidepressant properties that was unrelated to the benzodiazepines. While hardly a miracle cure, the nurses were convinced that it made a difference. An alternative explanation for Leyla's mellowing was tincture of time. With time, she came to believe that she was safe. She had to test the system—she had to call out at two P.M. and three A.M. to prove that the nursing staff was truly at her disposal. She had to test her family, who felt increasingly guilty about their decision to institutionalize her, so as to convince herself that they would continue visiting her, no matter how abominable her behavior.

Some days she called out so incessantly that her roommate could not stand it anymore. In a stroke of brilliance, the nursing-home social worker arranged a roommate swap: Leyla's new partner was totally deaf and regarded Leyla as a charming lady since she couldn't hear the ruckus she made. Leyla, in turn, put up with her roommate's banging of drawers and nocturnal trips to their shared bathroom. Perhaps she recognized she could not be choosy; perhaps she found the perpetual reminders that she was not alone reassuring. Leyla suffered from relapses—periods when her anxiety escalated and her neediness increased to immeasurable proportions. But for the most part, she found the structured existence in the nursing home helpful. She liked the routine, the predictability of her life. There was a grand piano in the main lounge that she played every day for a few minutes before supper. She would never be happy, but overall, the nursing home gave her, and her family, a peacefulness they had not known in years.

Coping with frailty almost inevitably requires making changes in one's environment. Of the four people whose stories I tell in this book, only Ben Frank managed to stay in his original apartment.

He did so by hiring an aide, for thirty hours a week, who cooked, shopped, cleaned, and provided companionship. His helper's upbeat attitude had a salubrious effect on his mood beyond the material support she provided. Ben was able to remain at home because he could take care of his personal needs and because he had the financial resources to pay privately for help. Both the progression of his frailty and the dwindling of his money, however, made his staying at home increasingly tenuous.

Catherine Endicott made two moves: first, from the three-family house she had lived in for years to a one-bedroom apartment, and then on to assisted living. The first move was prompted by the deterioration of the neighborhood and the sheer size of her home. Maintaining a house was too much for her, and as all her friends died or moved away, there was little to keep her rooted. The second move was triggered by the anxiety of living alone with no on-site help in the face of recurrent medical problems. Catherine found she was increasingly calling either 911 or her daughters when she awoke in the night unable to breathe. She felt that if there were a nurse on the premises she might not need to make so many nocturnal trips to the hospital emergency room. Above all, she did not want to be a burden to her daughters, disturbing their sleep, causing them endless worry. She saw assisted living as an almost ideal mix of privacy and community, with the appropriate resources for frail older people readily available. She had as much, or rather as little, space as she had had in her apartment. She had three meals a day served in the common dining room, obviating the need for shopping or cooking, and providing her with social contacts during mealtimes. Just knowing that an attendant was available at any time of day or night and that a nurse would arrive each morning dramatically decreased the frequency with which Catherine called for help.

Free-standing assisted-living complexes such as the one

Catherine Endicott moved into have one major drawback: they offer no higher levels of care as backup in the event of short-term acute illness or during recuperation from a hospitalization or a fracture. A major motivation for Jack Simon's decision to move to a continuing-care retirement community was that it offered a continuum of services, including an affiliated nursing home. Initially, Jack was able to live independently, eating dinner in the communal dining room and availing himself of weekly house-keeping services. He knew that as long as his wife was alive and well, she would provide whatever additional assistance he needed. He liked the CCRC setup because it gave enough security to allow his wife to go off on her own periodically without having to worry about him in her absence. Its nursing home was on the premises, so that if either member of the couple needed more care, he or she would be able to get whatever was needed and still have his or her spouse close enough to spend time together.

When the care needs are very great, a nursing home may be the only practical alternative. Twenty-four-hour care is often prohibitively expensive, and many elderly people do not have the necessary physical space to hire live-in help. For Leyla Keribar, a nursing home offered an unparalleled degree of security. While even round-the-clock nursing care proved insufficient to assuage her boundless neediness, anything less would have been orders of magnitude worse. Leyla's tremendously caring daughter, who had done everything possible for her mother over a period of years, had become irritable and distraught when her mother had wakened multiple times during the night with hip pain. She would have burned out quickly had her mother stayed at home with her once she developed dementia on top of her Parkinson's and arthritis.

In addition to providing both physical care and much-needed reassurance, the nursing home served a social function. The other nursing-home residents were a source of companionship for

Leyla—some were equals with whom she could readily converse; others were people she could help since she was more cognitively and physically intact than they were. Recreational programs organized by the nursing home were another source of enjoyment for Leyla at a time when her impairments meant that trips to senior centers or the theater or concert hall were extremely difficult for her. For all the imperfections of a nursing-home environment, it provided the support necessary for Leyla as she descended further into frailty.

New types of living arrangements for senior citizens are appearing constantly. Assisted-living facilities have been created that focus exclusively on individuals with dementia. Providing care for people with memory impairment is a major challenge, since such individuals need reminders throughout the day rather than assistance in discrete packages. Continuing-care retirement communities have been developed on or near a college campus, to allow residents to take advantage of facilities such as a library or a gymnasium as well as cultural activities. Acute-care hospitals have formed relationships with CCRCs and assisted-living complexes to assure continuity of care for patients and to promote speedy discharge from the hospital. As the market has become more competitive, the nursing-home industry has become more responsive to the consumer. Nursing-home administrators draw on expertise from hotel management and restaurant management as well as geriatrics and gerontology to improve the quality of their facilities. The common theme in the many available living arrangements is that the environment matters. Safety and health matter, but so, too, do emotional and spiritual well-being. Family is critical and medical care is important, but community is essential for the frail to flourish.

CHAPTER 4

When Acute Illness Strikes

Patients today participate with increasing frequency in decisions about their health. The paternalistic model of the physician is in disrepute: instead of dictating to patients the course of treatment they must accept, physicians are expected to discuss options for care. They are to settle on an approach based on a discussion of the pros and cons of the various alternatives and the patient's personal preferences. While involvement in health-care discussions is appropriate for patients at every stage of adult life, it is particularly crucial for those who are frail. Young, healthy people who develop an acute illness such as a heart attack, pneumonia, or cancer will typically opt for whatever form of treatment offers the greatest chance of prolonging their lives. They are usually willing to put up with considerable discomfort in exchange for cure. While some elderly people make the same choices, many do not. They make different choices from younger, otherwise healthy individuals for three fundamental reasons: they are approaching the end of their lives, treatments may produce dependence and disability, and conventional treatment is less likely to succeed.

Claiming that age matters does not imply that patients should be denied treatment on the basis of age. Age is important simply because if you have a life expectancy of thirty years, you will probably accept two months of suffering, but if you have a life expectancy of six months because of your multiple chronic illnesses, you may find a two-month stay in an intensive care unit intolerable. *Some* frail older patients will take their chances with ICU treatment, either because they do not believe they are near the end of their lives or because they would accept any amount of discomfort in exchange for the possibility of life-prolongation.[1] They may accept aggressive interventions if they believe the only alternative is death, but if they are presented with an approach to care that is midway between comfort only and cure at all costs, they may be eager to forgo either extreme.[2]

Choosing how much medical care and what kind is particularly important for the frail elderly. People who have impairments in multiple domains and who already need help in many activities of daily life are at high risk of further decline from conventional medical therapy.[3] The person whose kidneys function well enough for him to get by from day to day but who has evidence of renal impairment on blood tests is at risk of developing drug toxicity when he is treated with antibiotics for an infection. The frail individual with borderline diabetes and chronic stable heart failure is likely to develop dangerously high blood sugar as well as fluid in the lungs from a simple case of the flu. The combination of multiple problems occurring simultaneously may so weaken her that she will need several weeks of rehabilitation before she can go home again. Hospitalization in an intensive care unit often causes acute confusion (delirium) in a frail person, which sometimes lingers for days or even weeks after the precipitating illness has resolved. Prolonged delirium usually cannot be handled at home, and is incompatible with rehabilitation, so it necessitates a nursing home stay.[4]

The final reason why frail older people face unique challenges when they become acutely ill is that standard medical care is often less effective for them than it is for their more vigorous counterparts. Old age by itself is not the issue—people in their seventies or eighties stand to benefit from contemporary medical know-how, including interventions previously denied on the grounds of age, such as thrombolytic therapy (clot-busting drugs) for a heart attack. Success rates decline, however, in those older people who have many coexisting medical problems. Either because the acute problem is more severe, and therefore harder to treat, or because complications are apt to develop (vigorous treatment usually depends on a working immune system, good circulation, and intact metabolism), a good outcome is less likely in the frail.[5] Unfortunately, physicians cannot state just what the odds are for someone with a particular set of problems—the eighty-five-year-old man with Parkinson's disease, diabetes, and emphysema, for instance, who is contemplating chemotherapy for a newly diagnosed cancer. In the face of uncertainty, making medical decisions is excruciatingly difficult.

Ben Frank, Catherine Endicott, Jack Simon, and Leyla Keribar all developed major, acute medical problems at various points during their period of frailty. Together with their families and physicians, they made different choices about how to proceed, ranging from maximally invasive treatment to pure palliation, with watchful waiting and intermediate-level care in between. Their decisions were shaped by the circumstances (the prognosis of the acute condition and the options available), their assessment of their quality of life, and their understanding of their overall condition.

Ben Frank

At the start of Ben Frank's fourth and lengthiest hospitalization for CHF, Susan visited him every weekend. Each Saturday morning she took the four-and-a-half hour train ride from Boston to New York, and on Sunday evening she made the return trip, arriving home at midnight, physically and emotionally exhausted.

Once it became clear to everyone that Ben was going to be sick for a long time, Susan picked up and moved to New York to be near him. She negotiated an arrangement with her employer whereby she did her work by computer and stayed in communication by fax and phone. Once every two weeks, she returned to Boston to do any work that absolutely necessitated her physical presence.

For two months, Susan's life revolved around her father. It was a time of great intensity for her. She became closer to her father, getting to know him in ways she never had. She called me frequently during that period, sometimes from Boston, usually from New York, typically to ask me to translate the doctors' lingo. I became her interpreter as she plunged into the world of bronchoscopy and feeding tubes and respirators. I came to see the tremendous difficulties inherent in letting go, both for family members and for physicians, in a new light. As a physician treating my own patients, I usually had strong beliefs about what was the right course of action for a given person; as a relative dealing with severe illness in my father-in-law, I likewise had had strong convictions about what constituted the right way to proceed. With Susan, I vicariously experienced the roller coaster ride: optimism alternating with despondency, joy followed by sadness.

The cycle began the way it so often did with Ben. His ankles swelled and he became short of breath. By the time he agreed to call his doctor, his lungs were filled with fluid and he had a dangerously low blood pressure. His doctor immediately hospitalized him with a diagnosis of worsening congestive heart failure, and transferred him from a regular medical floor to the intensive care unit when the seriousness of his condition became apparent.

Susan called me from the hospital during one of the many periods when she had been asked to leave her father's cubicle in the ICU so that he could "get care."

"Can he talk to you? Does he recognize you?" I asked.

"Yes and no. He knows me. He seems too tired to talk. He just says he wants to go to sleep."

"Did they tell you something about how sick he is?"

"They just said he has congestive heart failure and is getting heart medication."

"But there must be more going on if he's in the intensive care unit," I insisted gently.

"They said his blood pressure is low."

My ears perked up at this. "How low?"

"I don't know."

"Did they say he's had a heart attack?"

"They said he might have had a heart attack before he came in, a few days ago. They had to give him diuretics and then his blood pressure got really low. So they put him on some kind of strong medicine that he gets through a pump, just a few drops every minute."

Dopamine, I thought to myself. *He's on a dopamine drip because he's in shock.* Probably cardiogenic shock—profoundly low blood pressure due to a heart that just couldn't pump well enough. The mortality in eighty-three-year-old men with shock was high. Probably at least 30 percent. Maybe more like 50 percent.

"It sounds serious, Susan." I thought I heard her sobbing. I wished I were with her, to see her face, to reach out to her.

"I know it's not good. He's had heart problems before, but I don't think he ever had a heart attack. He was never really sick."

"At least he's better today," I said, not wanting to come on too strong. In addition, I did not have all the facts. It would be presumptuous to diagnose or predict based on incomplete information. But I had seen many, many frail older men go into the ICU, and not nearly as many come out. If they survived at all, they were typically far more debilitated than when they first became ill. "Well, keep me posted, all right?" I concluded.

For three days, I heard nothing. I could not reach Susan. She was never at her father's apartment when I called, and as long as her father was in the ICU, he would not have a telephone. When Susan finally phoned, she was very excited. "He's moving out of the ICU. He's doing much better. His blood pressure is normal without that special medication. He's going to be fine."

"That's terrific!"

"I'll be glad when he's in a regular room. In the ICU, I'm always in the way. When I stand on the left side of his bed, they can't reach his urine bag. When I go to the right side, they can't get to his intravenous. And when I stand at the foot of the bed, I block their precious clipboard, on which they record everything—each burp and each bowel movement."

"An ICU isn't a very friendly place," I concurred.

"And the lights are on twenty-four hours a day, with buzzers going off and nurses darting in and out to do things. Dad got totally disoriented."

"It's good that he's graduating."

But two days later, Susan's tune had changed. "They're so

understaffed, they don't pay any attention to him. He rings for the nurse to ask for help going to the bathroom, and no one shows up for half an hour. He can't wait half an hour. Once he urinated in his bed and they yelled at him, saying they were going to have to put a diaper on him."

I did not want to justify the nurses' behavior, but I empathized with their predicament as well as with his. "It sounds like he's a *lot* better if he's able to get up and go to the bathroom."

"I guess so." Susan sounded dubious. "He's very weak. The reason he has to call the nurse to go to the bathroom is that he is too wobbly to get up on his own." She paused. "He's also sort of confused. There's one nurse who is wonderful. She told me he had ICU psychosis. Some of the others treat him like he's two years old." Susan sounded sad and angry.

"If he's just confused from being so sick and, as you said, from being in the disorienting environment of the ICU, he'll get better."

"I hope so," she muttered as we said good-bye. This time I was guardedly optimistic, but Susan sounded discouraged. Perhaps it was just the transition from the ICU to a regular hospital floor. Despite all the disruptions in the ICU—the interruptions of the sleep-wake cycle, the sterile, artificial environment in which every movement was measured—the amount of attention was formidable. What was "intensive" about the ICU, more than anything else, was the nursing care. Moving to a conventional hospital floor was always a letdown. Each nurse looked after eight to ten patients instead of two. Though the ICU nurses were busy, they sometimes managed to find the time for a quick back rub. They spent so much time with those in their care that families experienced a powerful bond—even if the person the nurse got to know was only a pale reflection of his usual self.

Ben Frank did get better: his "ICU psychosis" cleared, and his congestive heart failure came under good control. But just when

Susan was tentatively thinking about returning to Boston, just when she began believing that her father had stabilized and was ready to embark on a course of intensive rehabilitation, he began developing low-grade temperatures. A chest X ray showed what was labeled a hazy opacity, and close comparison with his admission film—a poor-quality study done with a portable machine in the emergency room because he had been so desperately ill—suggested that the ominous shadow had been present all along. Ben's doctor asked a lung specialist to see him. The pulmonary physician was worried that Ben had lung cancer and advised a computerized axial tomography (CAT) scan of the chest. The CAT scanner, a big tunnel-like machine, gave inconclusive results. The pictures from the scan confirmed that something was in the right lung that didn't belong there, but did not elucidate its nature. The scan showed no enlarged lymph nodes adjacent to the unidentified substance, which was a good sign, since plump lymph nodes were often associated with a malignancy. But the absence of lymph nodes by no means implied that the mass *wasn't* a cancer. It could be tuberculosis, it could be pneumonia, it could be cancer, or it could be any number of more obscure diagnoses.

The pulmonary specialist recommended bronchoscopy, a procedure in which a tube is inserted through the mouth and into the lung. The physician peering in at the other end can actually see inside the major branches (bronchi) of the lungs. Any tissue pushing its way into the bronchus from the outside, or growing within the bronchus, can be biopsied and examined under the microscope.

"So Dad's going to have a bronchoscopy tomorrow," Susan told me.

"He is?" Why, I wanted to know. What were they looking for? What would they do with the information?

"The pulmonary doctor thinks it's lung cancer. But he says they caught it early and Dad could have radiation treatments." She sounded optimistic.

"Cancer? Radiation?" I was having difficulty imagining this. Ben Frank, an eighty-three-year-old man who had barely survived an exacerbation of congestive heart failure and who could not get out of bed by himself was going to get radiation therapy five days a week for a month or longer? Where would he live? How would he get to the hospital for the treatments?

More important, why? Why should he undergo radiation therapy, even if he did prove to have lung cancer? Radiation treatments could not cure lung cancer. Their major benefit was to ameliorate symptoms. But Ben Frank's only symptom was a low-grade fever. He was not developing recurrent pneumonias, he was not coughing up blood, and he was not short of breath. Radiotherapy would itself *produce* symptoms. For the duration of the treatment, it would cause fatigue—in someone who was already weak and exhausted. Given the location of the spot in the lung, there was a high risk of the radiation hitting the neighboring esophagus and causing chronic esophagitis. This is a sometimes debilitating condition that makes it painful to eat. And while the treatment sessions during which the radiation would be administered were brief and painless, they required daily trips to the hospital. If Ben was really on the verge of discharge, the last thing he wanted was to return to the hospital each day. The issues of discharge and of his underlying prognosis—even without a cancer diagnosis—were, I thought, central. At eighty-three, how much time did he have left? Did he want to spend the better part of the next month undergoing treatments that would cause more symptoms than they would cure?

"He's too weak for chemotherapy. I don't think his system could tolerate it. But I understand that radiation is pretty, well, mild," Susan explained.

"Comparatively speaking," I acknowledged. "The bronchoscopy is tomorrow, you said?"

"Yes, tomorrow morning." I could feel the pressure from Ben's physician to know, to diagnose, to treat. Ben Frank had entered the hospital because of congestive heart failure. He had survived, thanks to modern medicine, for which he and his daughter were deeply grateful. That same technological imperative that had saved his life was now driving his physicians to chase down an elusive shadow on an X ray. Maybe his doctors were right to keep pushing. "Dad's doctor says he's basically healthy—he has this congestive heart failure, and he has the trouble with falling that nobody can quite figure out. But other than that—and his hearing, of course—he's fine."

I didn't think he was fine, though there was no single organ system I could identify as the problem. He seemed to me to be frail and to have been progressively declining over the previous year. But perhaps I was overly pessimistic. Ben's doctors evidently did not think he was at the end of his rope, and Ben was eager to take whatever steps were necessary to keep on going. "Let me know what they find," I exhorted Susan. "Call me as soon as you hear." Maybe the real reason for proceeding was to be *certain* about what was going on in Ben's lung. For some people, uncertainty is worse than a cancer diagnosis. Uncertainty can produce paralysis of the will; with knowledge there is at least the possibility of action.

The results were surprising. "He doesn't have cancer!" Susan announced with evident relief. "But now they think Dad's having the low-grade fevers from a swallowing problem, and they are recommending a gastrostomy tube."

"I'm glad the cancer business was a false alarm," I said. "But why the rush to put a tube in his stomach? How long do they think he's been aspirating?"

"They don't know. But they did a special swallowing test—"

"A videofluoroscopy?" I interrupted.

"That's it. And they said every time he swallows solid food, a little bit goes into his lungs."

"And what do they think causes that?" Susan didn't know. "He could have had a small stroke somewhere along the line, affecting his ability to swallow. Or this could just be part of his generalized weakness after being sick and on medications in the hospital. If it's just a consequence of his being debilitated, then the fix is for him to get his strength back, not for him to have a tube."

"I'll ask why he has trouble swallowing," Susan indicated.

"And there's one more thing you should know. Generally speaking, gastrostomy tubes do not prevent aspiration. Maybe they decrease the likelihood, but even that's not clear. Food can reflux back up from the tube into the mouth and then go into the lungs. Also, people who aspirate regularly can get pneumonia just from aspirating their own saliva. A gastrostomy tube doesn't have any effect on that."[6]

"So, why would they propose a gastrostomy tube if it doesn't work?"

"Well, it's worth clarifying if the issue is neurological, based on a stroke. Then a tube may make sense just to facilitate eating, quite apart from the aspiration issue."

"No one said anything about a stroke," Susan insisted.

"Well, just ask about the basis for the aspiration."

"They're planning to put the tube in the day after tomorrow," Susan said. "They don't think it's such a big deal."

Just a minor procedure. Not a big deal. He'd been through the ICU, a dopamine drip, a CAT scan, bronchoscopy. Percutaneous endoscopic gastrostomies, or PEGs, as they are known familiarly, have revolutionized artificial feeding. Formerly requiring abdominal surgery, tube placement now can be done under local anesthesia, with sedation. First an endoscope is passed through the mouth and into the stomach, very much like a bronchoscope, but traveling through the esophagus instead of the trachea. Then the surgeon or gastroenterologist makes a small incision in the skin overlying the stomach, slides the permanent tube through the endoscope directly into the stomach, and passes the other end through the incision. Once the tube is secured, it can be used for nutrition. The plan in Ben Frank's case was to replace eating entirely, substituting tube feedings.

Susan was unable to find out the exact mechanism of the swallowing problem. But she did relay the doctor's conviction that aspiration was an ongoing issue and that the PEG, while not a guarantee against future aspiration, would lower the risk. In any event, Ben sailed through the gastrostomy tube placement. There was, however, one consequence of the procedure that had not been discussed: Ben would almost certainly have to go into a nursing home, and the level of care he required would be higher now that he was being fed by tube. Susan began the arduous and often disheartening process of checking out nursing homes for her father.

"At least I won't have to worry about him lying on the floor," Susan rationalized. "Or about Carmela not showing up, or about him running out of money. He's already eligible for Medicaid. I just have to finish taking care of the paperwork." She sounded tired, sad, relieved, and guilty all at once.

"You did everything possible to keep him out of a nursing home as long as possible," I assured her.

"I'm not sure whether to close up his apartment or to hold on to it, in case he gets well enough to go back."

I winced. Why did I feel as though I always feared the worst? "I don't think he's going to be able to go back home," I said, as gently as I could.

Susan sighed. "I suppose," she allowed.

Susan never had to choose a nursing home or decide what to do about the apartment. The following day, Ben Frank developed a massive aspiration pneumonia. He was transferred to the intensive care unit, to the same bed in which he had begun his hospital sojourn two months earlier. He again had an intravenous to deliver fluids, and a catheter to measure his urinary output. He again was put on a dopamine drip, this time for septic shock—profoundly low blood pressure caused by overwhelming infection. In addition, he was put on a respirator to help him breathe. For twenty-four hours, technology and vigilant nursing care sustained him. Despite all the tubes and the monitors, the medications and the attention, his respiratory status began to deteriorate. He developed an acute worsening of his congestive heart failure on top of the pneumonia. His blood pressure plummeted. His lungs, his kidneys, and then his heart gave out. Cardiopulmonary resuscitation was attempted, but, as is usually the case with frail older people, it failed. [7] Perhaps mercifully unaware of his surroundings, Ben Frank died.

Catherine Endicott

Catherine Endicott firmly believed that her heart would be the death of her. She knew that despite the angioplasty, several of the blood vessels feeding her heart were narrowed and one was totally blocked. She knew that much of the damage to her heart muscle was permanent, hence the long list of medications she took, including digoxin, a diuretic, potassium, an ACE inhibitor, and a beta-blocker. When she came down with the flu during her first winter in assisted living, and proceeded to develop shortness of breath, she figured it was her heart. This time Catherine did not panic. She knew what she had to do. She called the nurse who came daily to check on the residents of the facility. The nurse took one look at her and called Dr. Fields. In short order, Catherine was on her way to the hospital.

The physician in the emergency room also assumed the problem was her heart. Catherine could hardly breathe because her lungs were filled with fluid. She had pleural effusions—accumulations of fluid in the sac surrounding the lungs, a space normally filled with a small amount of lubricating fluid. A whole host of conditions could lead to the development of a pleural effusion: the most plausible in Catherine Endicott's case was congestive heart failure. When the heart did not pump strongly enough, blood backed up into the circulation in the lungs and the liquid component of the blood leaked out into the surrounding tissue.

Pleural effusions can be large or small; they can be in one lung or in both lungs. Catherine Endicott had effusions in both lungs—a small one on the right and a large one, occupying nearly half her lung, on the left. Lopsided effusions were a bit unusual in congestive heart failure, but not unheard of. The intern taking care of Catherine in the emergency room was not concerned about the idiosyncrasies of her case. He was too busy saving her life.

Catherine was struggling to breathe, but she was fully aware of what was happening. She felt the pain when the young doctor took a blood sample from the artery in her wrist to measure the amounts of oxygen and carbon dioxide in her blood. She heard the alarm in his voice when he reported the results: the oxygen was perilously low, and the carbon dioxide level was dangerously high. Catherine was in respiratory failure, and the only way to improve the situation reliably was to put her on a ventilator.

"I'm going to have to intubate you," the physician told her. "I have to put a tube down your throat and into your lungs and attach you to a breathing machine." He looked at her, uncertain of how to continue.

"Go ahead," she directed him. "Do whatever you need to."

The intern did not consider the situation any further. Intubation made medical sense. His patient seemed to be alert and to understand what he was saying. There wasn't much time. He urgently paged the anesthesiologist on call to intubate Catherine Endicott, simultaneously calling the respiratory therapist to hook her up to a ventilator. An hour after her arrival in the emergency room, Catherine had a catheter in her vein (to get medication), another catheter in her artery (to measure oxygen levels), a catheter in her bladder (to keep track of urine output), and a tube in her trachea (to enable her to get oxygen). She was wheeled to the medical intensive care unit (MICU), where she had electrodes placed on her chest to provide continuous monitoring of her heart, and a nasogastric tube inserted through her nose and into her stomach to provide nutrition.

With the ventilator controlling the most urgent problem, Catherine's breathing, the MICU physicians reviewed the data that had been collected so far. They went over the chest X ray that showed the pleural effusions, the white blood cell count that was strikingly normal, the electrocardiogram that demonstrated acute ischemia (possibly a heart attack), and assorted blood chemistries. Not satisfied that they had the full picture, the physicians proceeded with further tests. They stuck a large needle into the pleural space—the fluid-filled sac enclosing the lungs—and removed a pint of fluid to examine under the microscope and to send for special tests. They ordered more blood tests to ascertain whether there had in fact been heart damage. Finally, they prescribed a long list of medications and moved on to the next patient. The missing part of the evaluation was the history—Catherine Endicott could not speak because of the respirator.

Catherine recalled spending a sleepless night. Every half an hour a nurse checked her tubes or helped her turn in bed or drew yet another blood sample. The lights in the MICU were never turned off, and the chatter of the professional staff continued, unabated, throughout the night. Most likely Catherine dozed off periodically. Her daughters came to see her, were dismayed to find her with a tube in every orifice, stayed for the brief periods allowed in the MICU, and went home.

The pleural effusion results were perplexing. The fluid was an exudate, thick and viscous, as happens with infections and tumors rather than with congestive heart failure. The cytology report—the results of examining the fluid under the microscope to look for tumor cells or infection-fighting cells—was inconclusive. The cells were all normal-looking blood cells, mainly white blood cells of various types, but there were not enough of them to be sure a tumor cell wasn't lurking about somewhere.

While the pleural tap—the removal of the fluid—did not elucidate the cause of the fluid, it did serve to ease Catherine's breathing. Without all that fluid pressing on her lungs, Catherine was able to breathe on her own. Within a day, the ventilator was disconnected.

"How does that feel?" asked the intern who removed the tube.

"It feels wonderful. I can talk again."

"You're doing great. You didn't have a heart attack and we don't think you were in congestive heart failure."

"So why couldn't I breathe?"

"You had a lot of fluid in your lungs, which we removed."

"Fluid from what?"

"Well, honestly, we don't really know. We'll have to see how things go in the next couple of days."

Things did not go well. Within two days, the fluid had significantly reaccumulated. Within three days, Catherine was back on a ventilator. Once again, fluid was removed with a needle and syringe, and once again it was studied and tested. Once more, the fluid would not betray its origins. Dr. Fields presented Catherine and her family with the options.

"I think we have to get to the bottom of this fluid situation. And I think the only way we will be able to do that is by taking Catherine to the operating room and putting her to sleep. Then we can do something called a mediastinoscopy—we can actually get a sample of tissue right next to the lungs—and at the same time we can do a bronchoscopy—we can look down into the lungs. We can also completely drain that effusion, taking out every last bit of fluid, and do a pleural biopsy—get another piece of tissue from the lining around the lungs. Once the fluid is all out, we can inject a sclerosing agent, material that will effectively glue the two parts of the pleural sac together so that fluid cannot build up there anymore."

"How risky is this?" Jennifer inquired.

"Well, it is surgery. But it's not a very lengthy procedure. And your mother didn't have a heart attack this time. Actually, her heart's doing remarkably well."

"What's the alternative?" Jennifer pushed him.

"We could drain the fluid off and inject that material under local anesthesia. Then we wouldn't get the biopsy, so we might still not know what we're dealing with. And doing the injection under local is a pretty brutal business. Even with a lot of pain medication onboard, it's no fun."

"Anything else?"

"I would have said we could leave things alone, but if the fluid reappears in two days, that's not a viable solution. If it were every few months, that would be a different matter."

"What do you think, Mom?" Andrea asked skeptically.

Catherine was intubated again, so she could not speak. She tried writing a few words, but her scrawl was indecipherable.

"Are you willing to have an operation?"

Catherine nodded.

"Or would you prefer the smaller procedure?" Andrea continued.

Catherine shook her head.

"You understand you might get into trouble," Dr. Fields added, by way of trying to get informed consent. "You could have another heart attack from the stress of the operation. You could have bleeding complications or get pneumonia afterwards. And you could die. Though," he added hastily, "I think that's very unlikely." Catherine shrugged, as though saying that what will be will be.

A day later, Catherine Endicott was admitted to her second intensive care unit, the surgical ICU (SICU). She got through the procedure without any problems and was transferred to a regular floor, where she began the slow, arduous process of recovery.

Five days later, just after she had begun walking on her own, her lungs filled up with fluid again. This was a different kind of fluid. Instead of filling the space outside the lungs, this fluid was in the air sacs themselves. This fluid was classic pulmonary edema, due to a failing heart. It was treated with high doses of diuretics. Because she was acutely ill, Catherine was transferred to her third intensive care unit, the coronary care unit (CCU).

Dr. Fields couldn't say why Catherine had tolerated the stress of surgery only to develop heart failure several days later. Again he checked for a heart attack—negative. Perhaps attempting to walk had tipped the balance. This time her congestive heart failure was so severe that she was put back on the respirator. Every time her breathing improved and she seemed not to require the machine, her failure got worse again. After extensive tinkering with her medications, Catherine began to get better and the respirator was removed.

Each step forward, Catherine commented, was followed by at least one step backward. She survived the operation only to develop heart failure. And once her heart disease was under control and she was off the breathing machine, the diagnosis came back on the biopsy.

The pathologist had had to do all sorts of special tests on the tissue sample, but now he was convinced: Catherine Endicott had lymphoma, a cancer of the lymph glands. She was scheduled for a CAT scan of the abdomen to see if there was disease outside the chest. There was. Catherine was diagnosed with Stage IV non-Hodgkin's lymphoma.

"I never thought I'd get cancer," Catherine admitted to her daughter Jennifer. "I always figured all my problems were related to my heart."

Jennifer understood. They all had been so convinced that Catherine would die of her heart disease that they could scarcely believe she had lived long enough to develop another medical problem. "You'll fight this, Mom. The oncologist says the chemotherapy's not bad at all."

As chemotherapy went, that was true. Catherine would get Leukeran and prednisone. The prednisone could make her diabetic and potentially worsen her heart failure. Her treatment course was brief, just a few weeks, not long enough to develop osteoporosis or significant weight gain. After those few weeks, Catherine would remain on the Leukeran. Her white blood cell count would fall, but hopefully not to dangerously low levels. She might feel a little tired, but she would be otherwise asymptomatic. She could, of course, skip the chemotherapy and take her chances. The only symptom of the cancer arose from the fluid in the chest, and that problem had been treated with the surgical procedure. Chemotherapy was more preventive than anything else, intended not to cure the lymphoma, and certainly not to ameliorate symptoms, but rather to avoid future flares.

Catherine Endicott had always had modest expectations. She had been realistic when her husband had had a stroke, never deluding herself that he would be able to return to work and provide for his family. She knew after his stay at the rehabilitation hospital that from then on she would have to care for him and support her daughters. She had had modest expectations when she developed angina, once she realized what it was. She had refused bypass surgery because she thought it was hubris to undergo open heart surgery at her age. She was convinced that if she aimed too high, for cure instead of palliation, she could come crashing down, perhaps with a stroke, which she thought of as worse than death. So when the call came that their mother was intubated and in the intensive care unit, her daughters thought it was a mistake. They did not believe their mother would have authorized any such drastic measures. They assumed she had been pushed into accepting more aggressive treatment than she wanted. Had she been coerced? Or, when faced with imminent death, did she choose the only course that offered her life? Alternatively, did Catherine make her choice because she was not offered any relief other than the ventilator from the suffocating sensation she was experiencing?

When I met Catherine Endicott, as she struggled to get back on her feet in a skilled nursing facility after a one-month hospitalization, I asked her about her decision.

"I don't think I was worrying about dying," Catherine reflected, recalling the first of what would prove to be a cascade of high-tech medical interventions. "I just felt awful. I couldn't catch my breath. They gave me all kinds of medicine and I still couldn't breathe. Then this nice young doctor told me he could hook me up to a machine that would breathe for me. I was tremendously relieved." Catherine paused, trying to remember just how she had felt. "I know exactly what the doctor looked like. He looked like a kid to me. He must have been fresh out of medical school. He had a little beard and a little mustache—I think he was trying to look older." She smiled. "He saved my life."

"So you're glad they went ahead and put you on a breathing machine?"

Catherine nodded. "This wasn't the same as open heart surgery. I was drowning in fluid. If that doctor had offered to kill me to put me out of my misery, I probably would have said yes to that, too."

"And if they had suggested another alternative, giving you morphine to relax you and then removing the excess fluid—do you think that might have been a reasonable approach?"

"I wasn't in any condition to think about choices. The quickest relief, that's what I wanted."

"Do you have any regrets now? You've been through so much—over a month in the hospital, half of it in intensive care units."

"I'm not sure," Catherine told me quietly. "I'm so weak now. I can't do anything for myself. I have to ask for help all the time. And I have cancer, too, you know."

I decided not to push her any further, though I wanted very much to know whether she would favor intubation again, should she develop new problems with her breathing. That question would have to await a later visit. I had stirred up enough for one day.

When I brought up the subject of intubation at a later visit, Catherine clarified her views. "It wasn't so bad. I couldn't speak with the tube in, and that was frustrating. But my daughters kept reminding the doctors that I could understand. So they told me what they were doing, they explained things to me. They asked me whether I had pain, whether I was uncomfortable. Answering yes-no questions was easy. Sometimes, if it was very important, or if I needed to explain something to them, I wrote down what I wanted to say. My writing was kind of shaky, and it was especially hard to write when I had all kinds of intravenous devices in both arms, but I could usually make myself understood."

"You were persistent," I observed. "And you had two advocates in Jennifer and Andrea."

Catherine beamed. "They were wonderful. They came every day. Both of them. They kept the doctors and nurses on their toes." *I bet they did,* I thought to myself.

"It sounds as though you would be willing to put up with a respirator again—though I hope it won't ever be necessary to consider," I added.

"It depends. I wouldn't want something like that just to keep me going. I wouldn't want to be a vegetable. I wouldn't want to have to stay in a place like this forever, either. I want to be independent. If I have a reasonable chance of getting back to where I was—back to the assisted living, where I have my own apartment and just need a little help—then it's worth it."

Jack Simon

Margaret Simon was convinced her husband had had another stroke. A year earlier, when *he* believed he had had a stroke because his vision was blurred, she had known better. On that occasion, she had been certain he had an eye problem and not a brain problem. Margaret had scoffed when her husband worried that he would have another stroke if he underwent surgery—she had been confident that he was unlikely ever to have another stroke. But now, she was not so sure. He woke up in the morning after an uneventful night with slurred speech. When Margaret could make out the words, she found he did not make much sense.

"My toopaysht is empsee," Jack said. Margaret finally decided that "toopaysht" was *toothpaste* and not *toupee*, primarily because he did use toothpaste but did not wear a toupee. "Empsee," she felt, was *empty*, but the sentence "My toothpaste is empty" was nonsensical. There was plenty of toothpaste in the bathroom, Jack had not yet been to the bathroom, and he seemed to be referring to a part of his body.

Margaret's certainty that she was dealing with a stroke increased further when Jack tried to get out of bed and found that his right leg was too weak to stand on. He had never regained full strength in that leg, and could not walk well, but he had been able to transfer—to get from the bed to a wheelchair and from the wheelchair to the toilet and to go short distances on foot. That morning, when he swung his legs off the bed and tried to stand, he collapsed. He fell onto the carpeted bedroom floor, managing not to hurt himself but unable to get up. At six feet and two hundred pounds, he was well beyond Margaret's lifting capacity. She tried to maneuver him so that he could get onto his knees and then stand, but he did not seem to understand what she wanted him to do. After half an hour of coaxing and coaching, pushing and pulling, Margaret gave up and dialed 911. Within minutes, an ambulance arrived. Two strong young paramedics hoisted Jack onto a stretcher, loaded the stretcher onto the ambulance, and transported him into the nearest hospital.

The emergency room physician also thought Jack had had a stroke. His blood pressure was up, his heart was racing, he could understand only a little of what was said to him, and he could speak less. While he was waiting his turn to go for a CAT scan of the head, routine blood tests were drawn. Surprisingly, his white blood cell count was markedly elevated at 20,000, suggesting though not proving that he had an infection. His temperature was taken hastily, and he proved to have a fever of 102. The intern remained convinced that Jack had had a stroke and speculated that either he had aspirated—food had gotten into his lungs as a consequence of the stroke—or he simply had had a "stress" reaction to the neurological event. The flaw in the first argument was that he had not had breakfast yet, making aspiration very unlikely. The flaw in the second argument was that the magnitude of the fever and the kind of white blood cells that were found were uncharacteristic of a stress response. A chest X ray failed to disclose a pneumonia and, even more interesting, the CAT scan did not show a new stroke. However, CAT scans can be misleading during the first day or two after a stroke, when the changes in the brain tissue that are picked up by a scan may simply have not yet occurred. The negative scan, the high white blood cell count, and the fever did not prove Jack *hadn't* had another stroke, but they pointed in another direction.

The other direction was the bladder. Jack's urine was cloudy in appearance. A drop placed on a microscope slide revealed it was loaded with white blood cells, and a special stain of the urine showed plump pink bacteria. Jack Simon was diagnosed as having a bladder infection, possibly even a kidney infection, a more serious illness typically associated with higher temperature, back pain, and sometimes shaking chills. The physicians prescribed intravenous antibiotics and admitted Jack to the hospital.

Twenty-four hours later, Jack's temperature was down to normal, his speech was clear, and his thinking was lucid. Equally impressive, he was back to baseline in terms of his strength. Jack's attending physician revised the diagnosis from stroke to urinary tract infection. A day later, he was switched from intravenous to oral antibiotics and discharged home. The doctors explained to Jack and Margaret that occasionally an acute illness masquerades as a stroke because the old deficits are transiently more pronounced. This phenomenon commonly occurs in diabetics who have an insulin reaction—their blood sugar becomes too low, they develop confusion, and, if they've had a stroke in the past, their weaknesses are exaggerated. Other illnesses, such as infections of various kinds or even heart attacks, can also manifest themselves without any telltale symptoms—just with confusion or strokelike signs. The reminder of how badly off he had been when he first had a stroke was sobering; the realization that this time he had escaped with a mere bladder infection was tremendously reassuring.

When the medical intern who was caring for Jack figured out that his patient had a urinary tract infection, he immediately recognized that what had made him prone to developing an infection was an enlarged prostate. Starting in their mid-forties, most men begin developing benign prostatic hyperplasia (BPH), and by the age of eighty, virtually 100 percent of men have significant BPH.[48] The intern performed a rectal examination on Jack Simon and satisfied himself that his prostate was palpably enlarged. He also thought he detected an irregularity of the surface rather than simply a smooth, generalized enlargement. Being a compulsive young physician, and aware that prostate cancer was common in older men, the intern sent a blood sample to the laboratory to measure the prostate specific antigen (PSA), which was typically elevated in prostate cancer.

Two days after being discharged from the hospital, Jack got a phone call from the intern. He began as though he were merely making a routine follow-up call to check on his patient. "Mr. Simon? Dr. Langston at Rivers Hospital. How are you feeling?"

Jack knew all too well that harried interns did not customarily make follow-up calls. "I'm doing great. What's up?"

"Well, one of your tests came back today. The PSA. I ordered it to work up your prostate. You know, we talked about how your prostate was a little large and that's probably why you got a bladder infection."

"And?" Jack had read about the PSA test in the newspaper, and was a bit annoyed that he had not known he had had one done while he was in the hospital.

"Well, it's kind of high. Not *very* high," he hastened to add. "But high enough that you should have follow-up."

"How high is it?"

"Twelve. Twelve-point-five, actually." That was the easy part, quantifying the test. The hard part was interpreting it. "Up to four is pretty much normal. Four to ten is borderline. Over ten is kind of high. But people with BPH tend to have higher PSA levels, so twelve could be normal."

"I see," Jack said, though he didn't see. As far as he could tell, the doctor on the phone was telling him he probably had prostate cancer. "I'll be in touch with my regular doctor. Thank you for calling." He hung up, sat motionless for a while, and then rolled his wheelchair into the living room to listen to the radio until Margaret returned home from her errands.

He could not concentrate on the radio program. Margaret found him sitting by the window, watching the world go by, the world that seemed to be filled with vigorous, healthy people. None of them appeared to have had a stroke, and they all seemed to him to be too robust to have cancer.

"Well, Margaret, the other shoe fell." Margaret was mystified. "We thought I was lucky that I didn't have a stroke—all I had was a bladder infection. Now it looks like it's cancer."

"What are you talking about?" Her first reaction was that he had been brooding again, like the time he mistook his cataract for impending doom. Jack explained—the phone call, the intern, the PSA.

"He tried to be matter-of-fact. He said it *might* be normal. But I could hear in his voice that he didn't think so. He thinks I have prostate cancer. Remember Len Wolf? He died of prostate cancer. Had it in the bones. It was terribly painful. Went on for months."

Margaret remembered Len Wolf well. He had been their neighbor for many years: their children had grown up together. He had been a busy salesman like Jack until his back began acting up. He thought it was a pulled muscle from playing tennis. He took so much aspirin for his back that he developed a bleeding ulcer. While he was in the hospital because of the ulcer, he had back X rays. The X rays showed he had metastases up and down his spine. He got hormone injections, which helped for a while, but then he just faded away. He lost fifty pounds in a couple of months. Margaret remembered visiting him during the last week before he died—he had been emaciated and on morphine. The morphine had controlled the pain reasonably well, but had left him groggy. Margaret shuddered involuntarily when she looked at Jack, imagining him wasted and weak.

"Let's not jump to conclusions," Margaret urged. "He didn't *say* you had cancer. He said you had an abnormal blood test. And I would remind you that this was the guy who also said you had a stroke, which wasn't true either."

Despite her arguments to the contrary, Margaret secretly suspected that her husband did have cancer. She had been thinking a great deal about death lately, perhaps because one of her closest friends had just died. Jack was eighty-three and she was eighty-one, and their friends, one after another, had been coming down with what would prove to be their final illness. Several had been diagnosed with cancer, a few had Alzheimer's disease. Her friend

Jocelyn had had a massive heart attack and died without warning. The funeral had been a week ago, just before Jack's hospitalization. Margaret had been too preoccupied with her husband's illness to grieve very much, but once he seemed to be all right, she had been struck by the loss. Margaret and Jocelyn had been friends for thirty-five years. They had met when they were both suffering from empty nest syndrome—their youngest children were off at college and they suddenly felt superannuated. Together they had carved out new careers for themselves: Jocelyn as a photographer, Margaret as an antiques dealer. They had shared each other's successes and disappointments, personal and professional. When they called each other on the phone it had been like two adolescent girls unburdening themselves—without the cattiness or jealousy or rivalry that sometimes marred teenaged friendships. Now Jocelyn was gone and Margaret felt an overwhelming loneliness. She had been wondering who in her circle of friends would be next and what her own fate would be when Jack sprang the PSA report on her.

Margaret kept her fears to herself, scheduled an appointment for her husband to see his primary-care physician, and waited. The appointment, she assumed, was likely to bring bad news. But at least it would bring a resolution to their uncertainty.

The Simons left the doctor's office in a daze. Their heads were swirling with information about "false positive tests" and "watchful waiting." Apparently it had not been such a good idea to order the PSA test. But now that it had been done, and it was abnormal, they had a choice. They could wait to see if symptoms developed, gambling that some other lethal problem was likely to come along before the prostate cancer spread—if Jack had cancer at all. Alternatively, he could have a biopsy done to determine if there were any detectable tumor cells in the prostate. If there were, he could still opt for watchful waiting, or he could have surgery. Surgery, if that was the route he chose, might leave him impotent and incontinent.[9]

Jack consulted a urologist, but he had the distinct impression that the doctor was procedure-happy. He spoke rhapsodically about doing a biopsy and became euphoric at the prospect of repeating the biopsy on an annual basis if it was negative. If it was positive, of course, that would mean an operation. A *big* operation. But, the urologist assured them, it was an operation he was really good at performing. There was the radiation-therapy alternative to surgery, which sounded as though it would be less invasive, less risky. It was true that the *mortality* was lower with radiation than with surgery. But radiation was more likely to cause sexual and bladder dysfunction. It also tended to produce problems with diarrhea. Severe, sometimes uncontrollable diarrhea.

"And what do you recommend for me?"

"We need to do a biopsy, and if it's positive, I'd favor a radical prostatectomy."

"What if you didn't operate?" Margaret asked.

The urologist looked puzzled. "Even though the biopsy was positive?" Margaret nodded. "Well, you could have radiation, though, as I said, it actually causes more problems than surgery."

"No, I meant what if you don't do either?"

"Do nothing?" the urologist repeated, incredulous. Margaret nodded again. "Well, eventually, most people go on to develop metastatic disease. That usually means the cancer involves the bones, which is very painful. It can also cause spinal-cord compression if it gets into the bones of the spine, which means paralysis."

"But does that always happen?" Margaret persisted.

"No, it doesn't," the urologist admitted. "And we're not yet very good at predicting in whom the cancer will spread."

"And how long does it take from having a small, localized tumor to getting bone metastases?"

The urologist acknowledged that the time was highly variable. "Could be months, could be years."

"Jack's eighty-three," Margaret said simply. She thanked him for his advice, rolled her husband out of the office, and asked the secretary to let the chair-car company know they were ready to go home.

"You're amazing," Jack told his wife once they were safely in their own apartment. "How did you know to ask all those questions?"

Margaret beamed at the praise. "I read an article about PSA screening in the paper. It's quite controversial. In Canada they don't do it at all. And I don't think many people recommend it for men in their eighties." [10]

"So, you don't think I have prostate cancer? Or you think if I do, something else will get me before I have any trouble from the prostate?"

"I'm not an expert. What I think you have or don't have is beside the point. Also, your situation is complicated because the test wasn't exactly a screening test. You had a problem from your prostate—you had a bladder infection, which they think is related to an enlarged prostate. The intern examined you and thought your prostate was abnormal, so that's why he ordered the test. Of course, the attending physician didn't feel anything alarming, so I'm not sure whether the PSA was a screening test or a test because of a strong suspicion you had cancer." She took a deep breath. "What I do think is that you need to see a different urologist. One who isn't quite so enthusiastic about cutting."

Jack agreed. He also spoke to his son Stuart, who volunteered to download all kinds of relevant material from the Internet.

Within a few days, he and Margaret had a thick envelope of articles to study about PSA and prostate cancer. It was a good project for him—motivated by a personal dilemma, but intellectually fascinating, something to sink his teeth into. By the time he had his appointment with urologist number two, Jack felt as though he were going in for a final exam after an intense period of studying.

"What it boils down to in your case," Dr. Seltzer concluded, "is how much uncertainty you are willing to tolerate. For some people, not knowing whether they have cancer is so anxiety-producing that they're better off finding out even if they wouldn't accept treatment." He let that register. "And also, even if you have cancer and you choose not to have surgery or X-ray treatments, there are other approaches besides doing nothing."

"Like what?"

"Like monitoring the PSA every six or twelve months to see if it starts going up, with the idea of intervening if it looks like the cancer is starting to cause mischief." Margaret frowned: she was not sure she liked the image of prostate cancer as a naughty imp, though she did find it less sinister than the previous urologist's caricature of the cancer as a wily and malevolent alien. "Or some people do well simply by lowering the level of testosterone, whether through an orchiectomy or by giving hormones."[11]

Jack cringed at the prospect of surgery to remove his testicles. "You mean you'd turn me into a woman?"

"Hardly. You'd still be very much a man. Your adrenal glands make testosterone, too, not just the testicles. But hormonal manipulations appear to lengthen the time until prostate cancer metastasizes."

"So it would be a race to the finish," Margaret interpreted.

Dr. Seltzer agreed. "When we do autopsies on men over eighty, a phenomenal number of them have evidence of prostate cancer. In most of those cases, the men were blissfully ignorant of the diagnosis, and in the vast majority, the cancer hadn't spread outside the prostate."

"I don't think I can decide this today," Jack said suddenly.

"That's fine. Why don't you go and think about all this, digest what we've talked about, and let me know what you conclude. If you want to come back in and talk some more, we can do that. If you figure out what you want to do, you can give me a call." He ushered the couple into the waiting room and shook their hands.

"I liked him," Margaret said simply after he had retreated into his office.

"I did, too, except I wish he had told me what he would advise."

"He felt he didn't know you well enough to be able to tell what would make sense for you. I did get the feeling that he thought watchful waiting would be okay. I also got the impression that if you do have a biopsy and it is cancer, you should opt for one of his intermediate strategies."

"But not that—that operation," Jack said lamely. They were both silent for a while. "I don't think I'm going to be able to sleep at night if I don't know what's what," Jack resumed. "You remember how anxious I was about the cataract surgery—wondering if it was going to be a success? I think I will be a nervous wreck if I don't have that biopsy. Every time my back acts up—and I do have a touch of arthritis—I'll be convinced it's metastatic prostate cancer."

"But if you do have cancer and you get back pains you'll be just as worried. Certainty only helps if the biopsy is negative. And then," Margaret mused, "you can worry about whether it was a false negative. After all, they just take five little samples, pretty much at random if there's no lump to biopsy, so you could have cancer and they could miss it."

Jack had reached a decision and was not about to be diverted from the course he had chosen. "If it's negative I'll be relieved—

even if I shouldn't be. And if it's positive, I'll take hormones or whatever Dr. Seltzer suggests."

The biopsy itself was uncomfortable but not intolerable. The hardest part of the procedure was trying to maneuver Jack onto the examining table with his weak leg. An ultrasound probe was used to visualize the prostate and identify any possibly suspicious areas. Five times, a long needle was pushed into the prostate and a small sample of tissue extracted. Then came two days of waiting (plus a good deal of soreness and some rectal bleeding), and, finally, the phone call. "Dr. Seltzer would like you to come in to review the biopsy results." Margaret and Jack knew immediately what that meant. A negative result could be given over the telephone. Only a positive result necessitated yet another office visit.

"I guess it came back cancer," Jack began.

"I'm afraid it did," Dr. Seltzer responded.

They reviewed the possibilities again. The urologist led them through the decision process. First he established that urinary incontinence would be devastating for Jack, who already had ample difficulty with washing and dressing. To have to wear a diaper and to have to change clothes more than once a day would interfere sharply with his independence. Next he found out that Jack's stroke had not rendered him impotent and that sex with his wife, though challenging because of his right-sided weakness, was an important part of his life. Dr. Seltzer also explained that a radical prostatectomy was a serious operation—quite apart from its possible side effects—one that he did not encourage eighty-three-year-old men to undertake.

"So, it sounds like hormones or wait-and-see," Margaret concluded. They debated these two alternatives.

Jack asked, "If hormones mess up the sex and I stop the hormones, will I be okay again?"

Dr. Seltzer smiled and nodded. "It may take a while for everything to settle down again, but yes, the side effects should be reversible." That clinched it.

"I'll try the hormones. I'll gamble that they will keep the cancer at bay. But if they cause more problems than they're worth, I'm going to stop." They had a deal.

The first few months were tough. Jack felt as though he were on trial whenever he reached for Margaret in bed. Periodically, as he had anticipated, he had a sharp pain in his back and became convinced that, as he said to Margaret, "This is the big one." After a couple of false alarms—both in bed and in his back—he stopped worrying and concentrated on his life.

Following a year of hormones and stable PSA values, Jack volunteered to help men work through "the PSA decision" as a member of a prostate cancer support group. He felt it was a natural extension of his work helping canned executives find new jobs: You started with the facts, then moved on to what mattered most to them. Then you looked at each option in turn and asked what consequences it would have. He was good at it. He liked talking to other men who were struggling with the same issues he had faced. He liked the fact that they typically found him a great deal less intimidating than they found their urologists. He enjoyed being living proof that more wasn't always better. He was tickled pink that having prostate cancer had given him a useful new occupation.

Leyla Keribar

During her first two years in the nursing home, Leyla's Parkinson's disease gradually worsened and her arthritis proved to be a chronic mild annoyance. But only once did she develop an acute medical problem. She complained of abdominal pain and was feverish.

When I went to see her, she looked ill—not deathly ill, but sicker than I had ever seen her. She was pale, her parkinsonian tremor was far more pronounced than usual, and she was confused.

Acute confusion, or delirium, can be triggered by any illness. After the stress of a hip fracture, for instance, as many as 44 percent of older people become transiently confused.[12] For those patients, like Leyla, whose baseline condition is confusion, as a result of a dementing process such as Alzheimer's disease, delirium makes them even more confused than usual. They may be agitated and noisy, or lethargic and apathetic. Frequently, their mental state waxes and wanes, so they may alternate between agitation and lethargy, with moments of lucidity interspersed. Infection, whether due to pneumonia or in the urinary tract, whether bacterial or viral, is commonly associated with delirium.

Whatever was giving Leyla a fever and abdominal pain was also making her delirious. As a result, she could provide very little by way of a description of her symptoms. I had to rely on information from the nurses, on my physical examination, on laboratory tests, and on statistical information about the most likely causes of fever and abdominal pain in women in their eighties. The nurses told me that Leyla had not vomited and that she had moved her bowels; physical exam confirmed that the problem was localized to the abdomen, mainly the left lower quadrant, and that there was no sign of obstruction from a twisted loop of intestine or a tumor. Blood tests pointed to the presence of an infection, almost undoubtedly bacterial. An X ray of the abdomen supported the clinical impression that this was not a bowel obstruction. My conclusion, putting all the data together, was that Leyla had diverticulitis, an inflammation of the small outpouchings of the intestine known as diverticuli. The treatment was to give the bowel a rest by substituting clear liquids for regular food, and to prescribe antibiotics.

Within forty-eight hours, Leyla was much better. Her temperature was back to normal, her pain was less intense, and she was more like her usual self. It would be a month before the delirium fully resolved, however, and with increased confusion came increased neediness.

Leyla was in some ways a vigorous woman. She had a strong heart, fine lungs, and normally functioning kidneys. Her problems were mainly with her brain: she had Parkinson's disease (a neurodegenerative disorder that affects gait and balance), she had mild dementia (a frequent concomitant of Parkinson's disease), and she had psychological problems. After her bout of diverticulitis, she suffered from gradual progression of her Parkinson's and slow deterioration of her thinking and memory. She did not develop any new, acute medical problems until she fell and broke her shoulder.

It was her right shoulder, and she was right-handed. The results were that she had difficulty feeding herself and brushing her teeth, and she could no longer dress herself in the morning. She could not play the piano, one of her few remaining sources of pleasure. She could not walk since she depended on a walker and was unable to exert the requisite pressure with her right arm. Instead, she was transported from place to place in a wheelchair.

In nursing home jargon, Leyla had become "total care." The only arena in which she remained independent was talking, and that she carried on with a vengeance. The calling out, which had abated for some time, resumed for hours at a time. It started early in the morning, when the night nurse was signing out to the day nurse, reporting on the new developments among her charges. "Nurse, nurse," Leyla would cry. The nurses would interrupt their transfer of information, and one of them would go to check on Leyla.

"What is it, Leyla?"

"I don't know."

"Do you need something?"

"No."

"Can I do something for you?"

"No."

"Margie will be in with your pills in a few minutes."

"Thank you," Leyla responded, unfailingly polite.

Five minutes later, the calls began again. Margie, the day nurse, asked one of the aides to go in to Leyla when she had a minute. She didn't really have a minute, since she was busy helping nine other residents get ready for breakfast, but when the cries became louder and shriller, she dropped by.

"Leyla!" she said, trying to keep the irritation out of her voice. "What's all the ruckus?"

"Ruckus?"

"You've been calling and calling. What's the matter?"

"I've been calling?"

"Don't you realize you've been saying 'Margie' over and over for the last ten minutes?"

"I suppose so," Leyla answered, somewhat dubiously.

"Well, Margie's busy but I'm here. What do you want?"

"Want? Nothing."

The aide shook her head. "Margie will be in shortly," she stated emphatically, and left.

So it went, for a good part of the morning. Margie sat with Leyla for ten minutes, trying to distract her from whatever unarticulated emotion distressed her. During those ten minutes, Leyla was lucid and appropriate. For perhaps fifteen minutes after the visit, she remained still. Then the calling out began again.

The staff brought Leyla into group activities: bingo games, arts and crafts, a current events discussion group. But Leyla was disruptive. She demanded personal attention. She raised her hand to answer a question during the discussion but then had nothing to say. Periodically she began calling "Help me, help me." At first the other residents were very concerned, insisting that staff tend to her immediately. When they realized she required no special help, they became less sympathetic. Some of them yelled at her to shut up as soon as the cries started. The social worker decided Leyla could no longer attend group activities.

The unit secretary wheeled Leyla over to the nurses' station and let her sit next to the phone. She talked to her between doing her paperwork and answering the phone. The strategy worked reasonably well, but some of the work conducted at the desk demanded greater concentration than was possible with Leyla sitting there making periodic remarks. Some of the work was confidential and couldn't be done with a nursing home resident within earshot. When her presence became too intrusive, the nurse escorted her back to her own room. She turned on the television; she had asked Valerie to bring in tapes of opera and encouraged Leyla to listen, wearing headphones. Every technique was transiently successful, but with Leyla's short attention span and endless neediness, only a full-time personal attendant would suffice to keep her calm.

Valerie did everything humanly possible, and more, to help her mother. She decreased her hours at work so she could come in every day to be with her. She spent upward of two hours straight holding Leyla's hand, talking to her, reading to her. On good days, Leyla seemed to be in a trance, under her daughter's spell, though she seldom recalled anything her daughter told her. On bad days, even Valerie's monologues were punctuated by her mother's cries for help.

"I'm right here, Mother. What is it?"

"Stay here, Valerie."

"I am here."

"Don't go."

"I'm not going anywhere." A pause. "Are you frightened, Mother? Are you worried?"

"No, I'm fine."

Valerie continued talking about her children, the concert she had gone to with George, news from Turkey.

I prescribed an increase in Leyla's Buspar. That made her groggy. She would doze off, only to awaken with a start to any passing footsteps and immediately call for help. I cut back to the previous dose of medication and asked the psychiatrist for advice. He suggested Ritalin, an antidepressant that took effect rapidly, unlike the traditional tricyclic antidepressants that took four to six weeks to kick in, or the newer serotonin reuptake inhibitors that had to be in the patient's system for at least two weeks before exerting any appreciable effect. I ordered Ritalin, a bit concerned that it might jazz Leyla up, since it is a stimulant, and believing that the last thing she needed was to be jazzed up. The drug produced no side effects, but it didn't help either. I increased the dose. Still no response. I stopped the medication.

Gradually, Leyla's fracture healed, and slowly, very slowly, she regained the use of her right arm. Her calling out tapered off slightly, but she continued to regress. Even when there was no clear physical explanation for her dependence, she required help with all the basics—the nursing assistants still had to bathe her, dress her, and feed her.

Because Leyla's overall condition had declined from near independence on entering the nursing home to near total dependence, I thought it was time to schedule a family meeting. The head nurse, the social worker, and I got together with Valerie and her husband to review Leyla's situation and discuss options for the future. Valerie and George were such involved family members that the reports from the various professionals about Leyla's status came as no surprise. Valerie had spent enough lunches with her mother to know she could not feed herself. She was in daily contact with her mother's primary nursing assistant and was well aware that her mother did not even select her clothes, much less put them on herself. She understood very well how exasperating care for Leyla could be—no matter how much you gave, no matter how much time you spent or how many special projects you came up with, you were not doing enough. Valerie was careful to acknowledge the frustration the staff felt, but her principal concern was her mother. Wracked by anxiety, unable to take care of herself, and progressively losing her memory, Leyla had little joy in life. Even Valerie's company and the occasional visits by her grandsons were only a partially effective balm, transiently ameliorating a fundamentally unpleasant condition. Valerie acknowledged that the previous six months had been immensely painful to watch. She wanted to know what the next six months were going to be like.

"Probably more of the same," I had to admit. "It's possible that Leyla will be more comfortable, paradoxically, as she deteriorates. Right now she is aware of her deficits. Her cognitive loss is still relatively mild, so she realizes, at some level, how much she has lost. Many people, as they become more demented, are no longer capable of understanding their situation. That can be a blessing." I stopped, not relishing pointing out to a family that worse could be better.

"So as she goes down hill mentally, she might become less anxious," Valerie summarized.

"Maybe." I couldn't say with certainty. "Each person is unique."

"She might also become more anxious, as she is less able to express what she feels and what she wants," Valerie mused. That possibility had crossed my mind. I nodded, acknowledging

Valerie's grasp of her mother's predicament. "So where do we go from here?" Valerie wanted to know.

"Well, I think we should try to keep her as comfortable as possible. And we should try to maintain the functions she still has—her hearing, her eyesight."

"Of course," Valerie agreed.

"We still need to discuss what to do if she gets sick. If, as her dementia gets worse, she develops trouble swallowing, would you want a feeding tube to maintain her?"

Valerie did not hesitate. "Absolutely not. Mother always said she wouldn't want to be kept alive as a vegetable."

"She wouldn't necessarily be a vegetable. She might well not be in a coma. She could be much the way she is now, except for the trouble eating."

"She still wouldn't want artificial nutrition. She told me that. 'When my time comes, let me go,' she always said."

"Different people have different ideas about how to define that moment." I was not trying to persuade Valerie to change her mind, but I did want to make certain she understood the issues.

"No tubes. I'm sure of that."

"So at this point, comfort is your overriding goal for your mother?"

Valerie agreed. "Her life is so awful! She never was like this. She was always active, vivacious, independent. She hates this existence. And I never imagined she would be reduced to this. She was always strong and capable." Valerie stopped and looked at me urgently. "Am I being cruel? Do I sound like a terrible daughter?"

"You're a wonderful daughter. You're incredibly devoted to your mother. And you're struggling to figure out what's best for her. You know her better than anyone else. I don't have any doubt that you know what's right for her." Valerie regained her composure. "That doesn't make it easy to decide what to do."

Valerie thanked me and asked one more question. "How much longer will this go on?"

"I don't know. Not too much longer," I said vaguely, responding as much to the pain in Valerie's eyes as to any medical data.

I was glad we had the conversation when we did. A month later, I was called by the nursing staff to see Leyla. She had a fever and had slept most of the day. She lay in her bed, breathing rapidly and coughing. This time she didn't have diverticulitis. She had pneumonia.

Pneumonia, "the old man's friend," as William Osler, one of the great American physicians of the early twentieth century, called it, is still a leading cause of death in the elderly.[13] On the other hand, many older people are successfully cured of pneumonia. In Leyla's case, there were several options for treatment. She could go to the hospital, where she would get intravenous fluids and antibiotics and could potentially be transferred to an intensive care unit if her condition deteriorated. I didn't think Valerie would favor that approach—it would be too traumatic for her mother. She could stay at the nursing home and receive antibiotics orally if she woke up sufficiently to take medications by mouth, or via injections if she remained too sleepy. Or finally, she could stay at the nursing home and be treated exclusively with comfort measures, using Tylenol to bring down her fever and oxygen to ease her breathing. I telephoned Valerie to update her on her mother's condition and to formulate a plan.

"Please, just keep her comfortable," Valerie implored.

"Of course. That's what we discussed."

An hour later, Valerie called back. "I'm sorry to disturb you," she began.

"You're not bothering me. What's up?"

"I talked to a friend of mine. She was shocked when I said

Mom had pneumonia and she wasn't getting antibiotics. She didn't think you could do that."

"What do you mean? Legally? Ethically?"

"Both. She thought Mom would suffer more and didn't think it was—it was acceptable procedure."

I decided to be very concrete. "Right now your mother's not suffering. Her temperature is near normal. She has plenty of oxygen in her system. And I gave her a little morphine to help ease her breathing. She's relaxed. More relaxed than she's been in a long while. I don't believe antibiotics would make her any more comfortable. If anything, over the short run shots would make her more uncomfortable. And over the long run—" I hesitated.

"Over the long run, are we killing her?"

"You aren't killing your mother, Valerie," I told her firmly. "And neither am I. She has lost her gag reflex—her ability to swallow food and to cough up her own secretions. Maybe antibiotics could help her get through this episode, though that's far from certain. But if they did, your mother would get another pneumonia in a week or a few weeks and the whole cycle would start over. Antibiotics can't fix the underlying problem. Your mother is dying, Valerie."

"I know." Valerie suppressed her tears. "I just had to make sure. People hear *pneumonia* and they think it's nothing. Just a little respiratory infection that pills can easily take care of."

"People who say that don't know what they're talking about. They don't understand." To successfully conquer pneumonia, patients require far more than antibiotics. They need a functioning immune system—white blood cells to attack the invading germs with antibodies and other white blood cells to devour the bacteria. They need adequate nourishment to have the energy to carry on. They need good circulation to be able to transport both antibiotics and the disease-fighting products of their own immune system to the battlefront. They must be able to swallow properly, both to take in sufficient nutrition and to ensure that the food goes into the stomach and not into the lungs. Leyla had problems with each of these functions. Antibiotics would do very little, if anything.

For three days, Leyla hung on. The first day, she was sleepy but could easily be awakened. She recognized Valerie, who was by her side most of the day. The second day, she was only minimally responsive, opening her eyes when Valerie called her name, but unable to process faces or words. By the third day, she had lapsed into a light coma. She moved reflexively when touched, but could not be aroused. She had not been able to eat or drink. She lay in bed, her heart still beating, her blood flowing, breathing rhythmically.

"She's gone," Valerie told me on the phone when we touched base. I was startled—the nursing home staff had not called me. "I mean her soul is gone," Valerie went on, sensing my puzzlement.

"You should go home," I suggested. "You've said good-bye. You need to rest." Valerie took my advice. At three A.M. that morning, I got the call from the night nurse.

"Leyla isn't breathing. She has no pulse."

I called Valerie. She knew what had happened as soon as the phone rang. "It's over," I said, meaning the agony of waiting as much as I meant Leyla's life.

"Oh, my God," I heard as she began sobbing. The finality was overwhelming. Before, there had been a hope; not a realistic hope, perhaps, but just the very slimmest hope that Leyla would return. Her spirit had departed, but perhaps the body that housed it would become well, and the spirit would reenter it. Now, all hope was extinguished.

The choices made by the four older people in this book when they faced acute medical problems ranged from maximally aggressive care to exclusively palliative care. Ben Frank accepted the approach recommended to him, which included a bronchoscopy for diagnostic purposes, a surgically placed feeding tube, and, ultimately, attempted cardiopulmonary resuscitation. Leyla Keribar, by contrast, was treated exclusively with comfort measures when she developed pneumonia. She got oxygen and Tylenol, but no intravenous fluids or antibiotics. Jack Simon opted for a course intermediate between these two extremes: when he was found to have prostate cancer, he selected hormonal therapy, not a radical prostatectomy.[14] Catherine Endicott fluctuated in her preferences, depending on the situation. When she had severe angina and was found to have blocked coronary arteries, she adamantly refused coronary artery bypass surgery, a major operation. As long as an option existed that merely involved medication, she favored the less invasive strategy. When she got repeated bouts of chest pain despite medication, she was amenable to a moderately invasive approach—angioplasty. Sometime later, when Catherine had a new problem—fluid in the lungs that made it hard for her to breathe—she was relieved to be intubated and go on a ventilator. Much later, when she became weaker and more debilitated, she chose to accept only those treatments available in the skilled nursing facility rather than undergo the disruptions and potential complications associated with hospitalization.

Why did these four individuals make very different choices about the type and extent of medical treatment when they were acutely ill? Might they have chosen an alternative approach if they had been informed of another strategy or if they had had a different understanding of their underlying situation?

When Ben Frank first entered the hospital in congestive heart failure, he was too sick to understand his situation fully. The oxygen level in his blood was low, making it difficult for him to think clearly, and he was having a hard time catching his breath, making him concentrate on the mechanics of breathing rather than the specifics of the physicians' treatment. Once he seemed to be recovering from the acute heart failure, his physicians were optimistic that he would survive and therefore believed that they should evaluate any and all abnormalities they detected, following each test with more tests until they identified and treated every problem. The physicians involved in his care almost undoubtedly did not think about Ben's underlying status. They addressed each of the series of problems he developed in the same way—as a puzzle that needed to be solved. They were driven by the impulses that drive most physicians—the desire to establish a diagnosis, and the wish for certainty. When Ben's chest X ray was read as showing a density that was possibly a tumor, the physicians were determined to elucidate the precise nature of the abnormality. If a chest X ray was not definitive, then they wanted to do a CAT scan. If the CAT scan did not yield an answer, then they proposed bronchoscopy. Their assumption was that the potential benefit of their tests outweighed any risks.

Geriatricians—physicians specializing in the care of the elderly—tend to be a bit more cautious. They are accustomed to accepting uncertainty, because they realize that the price of certainty is sometimes excessive. Knowing with certainty whether the chest X-ray abnormality was cancer might not be important if there was no possible treatment for Ben's lung cancer. Occasionally patients want to know what they have because, for them, worrying about what they *might* have may be more painful than the truth. Many patients are content to be observed—in the case of an X-ray abnormality, to have periodic follow-up, provided that there is no treatable problem that could be overlooked by failing to make a diagnosis. Geriatricians also tend to see procedures in a different light from other internists—not only as potentially likely to lead to complications but also as possibly inducing even greater frailty. For if a procedure does have an unfortunate outcome—for example, the sedation required to do a procedure may lead to the patient aspirating (developing pneumonia)—that outcome can then trigger a cascade of problems, delaying recovery.

Ben and his daughter, Susan, made the only choices they could have made, because they were not offered any other approach. Nor would the strategy of Ben's physicians have been unreasonable if Ben had been a robust older person rather than a frail person. Perhaps because he slid into frailty both quickly and insidiously, his condition was not entirely clear. In the face of ambiguity as to his overall prognosis, and given his perfectly clear will to live, his physicians advocated aggressive treatment.

Decisions about medical care in the frail, acutely ill person are family decisions. They intimately involve the physician, ideally a primary-care physician who knows the patient, and who should be able to discuss different options against the backdrop of the patient's underlying condition. If the physician has previously told his patient about her general health status and elucidated her goals for medical care, then he is in a good position to recommend a specific course of action. Though ultimately medical decisions rest with the individual, her physician and her family have crucial roles to play in figuring out what approach to take. Accepting and adjusting to frailty is a challenge for both the person who is frail and her family. In Catherine Endicott's case, her daughters initially argued for more aggressive treatment than she wanted. Over time, as they came to understand what frailty meant, the daughters were more leery of an approach they thought would leave their mother worse off over the short run, though perhaps better off over the long run, if she survived to experience the long run. Catherine, on the other hand, as she came to accept her limitations, found she derived meaning from life even though she needed a great deal of day-to-day help, and was willing to accept potentially life-prolonging interventions. Over time, as she felt herself nearing the end of her life, her priorities changed. Frailty comes in stages, and what makes sense during one stage is not necessarily what makes sense later on.

Jack Simon agonized over what course of treatment to pursue when he was found, quite accidentally, to have prostate cancer. The management of localized prostate cancer in octogenarians is controversial, and Jack and his wife were educated, thoughtful people who wanted to explore the options, so they sought out more than one opinion. Jack concluded that the high risk of impotence and incontinence made surgery a distinctly unappealing option, particularly since there was no proof that it would cure the cancer or even delay its spread. In his particular situation, there was a widely accepted approach to treatment that lay between surgery and comfort care. Hormonal treatment, together with ongoing monitoring for evidence of metastases, was an intermediate strategy that made sense to Jack.

Once Leyla Keribar entered the nursing home, the focus of her medical care increasingly became to maintain the functions she still had—enabling her to walk as long as possible and to participate in the few activities she continued to enjoy. As she became frailer, the goal of care shifted to ensuring her comfort. At first, treating potentially life-threatening illnesses such as infections made sense to her family, so when she was diagnosed with diverticulitis, I quite naturally treated her with antibiotics. Later, as her dementia became more pronounced and her quality of life deteriorated along with her mind and her body, her daughter felt that comfort alone should be the goal of care. As a result, when she had pneumonia, I gave her oxygen and morphine, allowing nature to take its course.

Other families might have drawn different conclusions about the approach to care. Religious values, for example, might have influenced them to accept antibiotics, arguing that prolonging life was a more important consideration than any assessment of the quality of that life. Even religious traditions that place a strong emphasis on the sanctity of life, however, typically do not insist on "heroic" interventions in a dying patient, nor do they require treatment that produces or prolongs suffering.[15] While another family might have opted for treatment if their relative was in Leyla's situation, at some point—perhaps after the second or third pneumonia—they might well have made the same decision.

CHAPTER 5

Not by Bread Alone

When I see patients who are old and frail, I cannot help but wonder what keeps them going, what sustains them spiritually as their bodies disappoint or betray them. My patients need ways to keep discouragement and despair at bay as they suffer the loss of their health, their independence, and, in many cases, their closest friends as well. To make matters worse, America's frail elderly live in a society that tends to devalue old age: fulfillment typically derives from work or raising a family, neither of which is a viable option for most frail older people.[1] A common way to deal with adversity is to focus on the bigger picture—on the meaning of life, on one's position in the greater scheme of things—a difficult strategy to invoke if the surrounding culture treats the frail elderly as having outlived their usefulness. What sources of satisfaction are available for older people in Western society today?

For the robust elderly—those who are chronologically old but are physically vigorous and cognitively intact—one source of gratification is pleasure. This is the proposed solution to the quest for meaning offered by the advertisers in *Modern Maturity*, the magazine of the American Association of Retired Persons. "You have worked hard all your life; now you deserve some fun" is the message, explicit or implicit, behind the ads for cruises to exotic islands, or fancy cars, or luxury condominiums on country club estates. Leaving aside the question of whether hedonism is ever the basis of fulfillment, world travel and upscale living are seldom options for the frail. Jack Simon could not get in and out of a car, whether a Cadillac or a Ford Taurus. Catherine Endicott relied on the sense of security she felt in the assisted-living complex and later in the skilled-nursing facility; she had no interest in residing, even temporarily, in hotels or guest houses, let alone in venturing to foreign countries.

Another possible path to fulfillment for older people is embarking on a new career, trying something you always wanted to do, such as playing a musical instrument or going into desktop publishing or opening a business.[2] This approach often requires greater initiative or talent or money than the average older person possesses. Frail older people might occasionally be able to carve out a new line of work—they may write their memoirs, or they may cultivate an old hobby—but for the majority, their physical limitations are simply prohibitive. Neurologic problems impede coordination, arthritis interferes with dexterity, macular degeneration adversely affects vision. Knitting or sewing, playing the violin or using a computer, are just not technically feasible for many frail individuals.

Compounding the difficulties inherent in finding meaning in life for frail older people is the reality that illness and disability often dominate their lives. Ben Frank was in and out of the hospital so often that he did not have much time to cultivate elevating pursuits. Catherine Endicott realized, when she moved into the assisted-living facility, that she spent hours every day on such basic activities as getting washed and dressed. She had to find meaning in the interstices of her existence: in brief encounters with other people, in occasional community meetings. Instead of concentrating on finding creative or stimulating ways to engage with the world, frail older people frequently devote their efforts to avoiding being "a burden" to their families. They seek independence, not the interdependence that is often the prerequisite for their participation in community life. Rather than taking the risk of spending their savings on a new endeavor, the frail focus on making ends meet. Though the elderly are financially in better shape than they once were, the image of the "greedy geezer" is a myth. Social security has been a great boon to the elderly, and old people are much better off with Medicare than they would be without it. But between the costs of medication, eyeglasses, and hearing aides, none of which is covered by Medicare, and the costs of nursing home care, which is seldom paid for by Medicare, the elderly spend $39 billion per year out of pocket for health care.[3]

There is no one strategy that frail people employ to enable them to cope with their condition and find meaning in their lives. The joys and the rewards experienced by Ben Frank, Catherine Endicott, Jack Simon, and Leyla Keribar are not readily generalizable. Their successes and failures, however, reveal several common threads. I asked Jack and Catherine directly about meaning in life, and I asked Ben's and Leyla's daughters their impressions of what sustained their parents. Relationships with family and friends and a sense of belonging to a larger community or culture were recurrent themes.

Ben Frank

Over a cup of minestrone soup in a casual Cambridge bistro, Susan talked about the last two months of her father's life. From my vantage point, many miles away from Ben Frank's hospital bed, the situation had appeared bleak. I had heard about the latest developments whenever there was a setback, a new problem, another trip to the intensive care unit. What I had failed to understand was how close Susan had come to her father in those stormy weeks.

"We were always close, but somehow we hadn't really *talked* in years," Susan explained.

I must have looked surprised. "For many years, while my mother was alive, she was the spokesperson for the two of them. She told me what she thought of my boyfriends and my jobs. She told me what she thought of my apartments and my painting. Dad was the quiet one."

"And after your mother died?" Susan's mother had been dead for a number of years.

"I guess he was out of practice. He wasn't used to saying what he felt. Or maybe he didn't want to be judgmental. Mom always had, shall we say, strong opinions. When Dad didn't say anything, I tended to assume it was because he agreed with her. But there was the possibility that he actually didn't agree, but that he preferred to remain neutral. When she was gone, he wanted to stay neutral."

"So, did you start talking again while he was in the hospital?"

Susan nodded. "I guess I'd been scared to ask him what he thought. Scared that if I could get him to express an opinion, I'd discover he didn't think much of me. I wanted him to think well of my work and my friends. I especially wanted him to be positive about my art. As long as he didn't say anything one way or another, I could believe whatever I wanted to."

I smiled. "It sounds like you decided to take the risk of finding out the truth."

"I'm not sure how it came up. I think I said something like 'Remember the time I was living with Roy, and Mom didn't approve?' And he said something like 'I remember, he seemed like a pretty nice guy. I always thought it was too bad that relationship didn't work out.' That broke the ice."

"Did you talk about art, too?"

"We talked about everything. After all, how many hours could we spend thinking about congestive heart failure and feeding tubes and other medical things?"

"I guess that's mainly what I talk about," I confessed. "At least with patients and their families."

"We talked about medical issues a great deal. But I was at the hospital for hours every day. We hadn't spent so much time together in years. Probably not since I came home for vacation when I was a college student."

"Was your father coherent enough in the hospital to really talk?"

"Not all the time. He was in and out. He had good days and bad days. Sometimes he was very befuddled and then suddenly he would come out with the most lucid comments. One day he asked for a painting of mine, something I had done, to have in his hospital room."

"Then you asked him what he thought of your artwork?"

"Actually, I was pretty cagey. I asked him which of my paintings he liked best, so I would know what to bring back for him the next time I went to Boston."

"And?"

"He told me he had never liked modern art, that he didn't understand it. And he said he didn't think I was very good at portraits, but he really liked my still-life work. The ones with pretty colors."

"Were you able to bring him a painting?"

"I did, but he decided he didn't want to keep it in his hospital room. He was afraid it might be stolen. I was so touched that he thought my stuff might be valuable enough that someone would want to steal it." Susan wiped away the tears. "He was a great guy," she managed to say.

"And if it hadn't been for those weeks in the hospital, you wouldn't have had all that time together."

"I wouldn't have given that up for anything," Susan told me.

"Did you realize how sick he was, that he might not make it?" I asked, a little nervous that this might be a sensitive area.

"Not at first. And even when I sort of knew—you made it pretty clear that the situation did not look good—I kept hoping. Whenever I thought he might not live, it became even more important to me to spend time with him."

"You were lucky that you figured out intuitively how to say good-bye."

"I never said good-bye," Susan responded sharply.

"I mean, you did all the things that the death-and-dying literature says you should do. You apologized for any pain you may have caused your parents. It sounds as though you gave your father a chance to say he was sorry for having offended you in the past. And you told him you loved him—in so many words."[4]

We stopped talking and suddenly became preoccupied with our now lukewarm soup. It was difficult to talk about dying. And just as the transition between robust health and frailty is often subtle, so, too, is the transition between being frail and dying. The duration of frailty is variable, but it always ends in death. Precisely because the frail person often does not have a single uniformly fatal diagnosis, families often do not appreciate how tenuous their relative's existence is and fail to prepare for death.

Ben Frank did not have a good death in the sense of dying peacefully and quickly, surrounded by his family, in the comfort of home. He might not have wanted to endure two stays in the ICU and a bronchoscopy if he had known with certainty that he would not survive the hospitalization. He would surely have preferred dying in his sleep to dying after an unsuccessful attempt at cardiopulmonary resuscitation, with a rib broken from vigorous chest compressions and a burn on his skin left by the paddles of the defibrillator. But given that neither Ben nor his doctor believed that the outcome of all the tests and treatments would be death, the effort made sense—and it gave him the opportunity to develop a special closeness to his daughter.

Did Ben Frank realize he was frail? Would an explicit acknowledgment of his frailty and its implications have made a difference in the choices he made during his final, two-month hospitalization?

"How did your father view himself during his last year?" I asked Susan as we moved on to coffee and dessert.

"He wasn't a very introspective sort of fellow, so I'm not sure he was terribly self-aware."

"Do you think he was discouraged by all his troubles—the heart failure, the falls, the inability to do things for himself?"

"The medical problems he more or less accepted. That is, I think he felt it was natural for his body to fall apart a bit. What he didn't accept graciously was medical help—not after his bad experience with the antidepressants that prevented him from urinating."

I was perplexed. "But he accepted all kinds of medical help in the hospital—both tests and treatments—didn't he?"

"Then he was scared. Also, he mellowed after his hearing got better. I think the single medical intervention that had the greatest impact on his life was the hearing aid."

"So once he could hear better, and interact more with people, he was much happier."

"I wouldn't say he was happy exactly, but he was reasonably

contented. When my mother died, he lost his raison d'être. He was no longer working. He didn't have any hobbies. He just withdrew further into his shell. When he adjusted to the hearing aid, and when he had that brief friendship with William—the man he met on the bench—he concluded that life was pretty good."

"And when he started to become frail, he still thought life was pretty good?"

"I guess so. Maybe it's a matter of your expectations. He didn't want to depend on others for anything—thank goodness for Carmela. She was the only person he would allow to help him. But other limitations he was able to accept—he didn't mind being able to do less as long as he didn't have to ask anyone else to do anything for him."

Dependence is what makes frailty so difficult for many people to endure. American culture values autonomy and self-reliance. We focus on the individual as the fundamental unit in society, rather than the family or the community, as in other countries and in other eras. The individual who can no longer be self-reliant, or who knows what he wants but needs others to help him realize his autonomy, tends to be disparaged.[5] Not only does our culture disdain the frail elderly, but the frail often see themselves as superannuated. This is in marked contrast to eighteenth-century America, for example, when older people were revered for their presumed wisdom. Attitudes gradually changed. As America became more urban and less rural, as the pressures increased for industrial employers to lay off older, less vigorous workers, the debilitated elderly were increasingly seen as a burden.[6] By the decade after the Civil War, the fundamentally negative attitude toward aging was firmly entrenched.

Expectations of what old age is like are intimately bound up with attitudes toward aging. As long as the expectation was that people would die in what is now considered middle age, anyone who survived into his seventies or eighties was considered remarkable. If his longevity was marred by disability, he was nonetheless strikingly unusual and worthy of veneration. As expectations changed, as a healthy old age became more and more common, the frail older person was increasingly held responsible for his predicament. Physical weakness was attributed to deficiencies in diet or exercise, and mental weakness was blamed on either too much or too little intellectual stimulation.[7] Today, the laudable *aspiration* to achieve a vigorous old age is sometimes confused with the *expectation* of disability-free final years. When frailty develops, often despite strenuous efforts to maintain health and strength, older people often feel they are failures, they are no good anymore. The wish "not to be a burden" that Ben Frank articulated is a common theme among the frail elderly. Catherine Endicott did not telephone her daughters when she had chest pain because she did not want to bother them. Jack Simon insisted that he and his wife move to a continuing-care retirement community because he thought it was too strenuous for his wife to take care of him in their own home.

Although the elderly try desperately to avoid calling upon their families for help, their spouses and children, paradoxically, often welcome the opportunity to help.[8] To be sure, caregiving can be physically exhausting and emotionally draining, but it can also be tremendously rewarding.[9] However, with the unprecedented mobility of American society, sons and daughters often live too far away from a frail parent to provide ongoing care. As an ever-growing fraction of the adult population works, there may be no relatives able to offer care. And as more and more people live into their eighties or nineties, a corresponding number of adult children are themselves elderly, and may be physically ill-equipped to serve as direct caregivers. Helping out—which may mean transporting a parent to medical appointments, doing the shopping, giving personal care, or arranging for all these necessities—is time-consuming and often anxiety-producing. Susan Frank was not exaggerating, however, when she said that the last two months of her father's life, time she spent largely at his side, was a gift. Frailty is not a condition any of us yearns for, but when it strikes, we need to accept it rather than see ourselves as failures.

Catherine Endicott

Catherine Endicott never got strong enough after her battle with heart problems and cancer to return to her apartment in the assisted-living complex. She remained in the nursing home and, in fact, moved to the section of the home reserved for the sickest, neediest residents. She became very thin, and the muscles in her hands and legs atrophied so much that she could walk only short distances and needed help dressing.

When I visited Catherine for a routine checkup, she was wan, thin, but elegantly dressed. I was struck by her dignity throughout her many illnesses. I was impressed by her resilience, by her sheer perseverance. I wondered out loud whether Catherine had had any clue as to what was in store for her. "You had plenty of experience dealing with chronic illness, taking care of your husband all those years after his stroke. Did you ever wonder what might happen to you when you got older?"

"Not really. There were too many grim possibilities. There was no point thinking about it. I just had to deal with whatever happened."

"But you did sometimes think about what it would be like to have a stroke."

"Oh, yes. I was terrified of having a stroke. That's why I didn't want to risk open heart surgery. Even though the chance of a stroke wasn't great, I wouldn't risk it. It's much easier to imagine having a particular condition if you've seen it up close, lived with it in your own family."

"Once you learned you had angina, did you have any sense of what the future would bring?"

"No. I don't think the doctors knew either."

"Did you do anything special to try to remain vigorous? To try to keep those blood vessels from getting any narrower?"

"You mean, like exercise?" I nodded. "Well, I was a very active woman. I figured that just in the course of cleaning the house, shopping, looking after my mother—when I first got the chest pains, my mother was still alive, you know—and going to work, I wasn't exactly sedentary."

"Sounds like you were quite a dynamo."

Catherine returned to my earlier question. "I don't think I changed my eating much. I did cut out sweets when I learned I was a borderline diabetic. And I always took my medication faithfully."

"You did very well for fairly long periods of time between heart attacks or episodes of angina or congestive heart failure."

"I was lucky. I was always a lucky woman." I found it hard to regard as lucky someone whose husband had had a stroke at forty, who had had to raise her children on her own, and who lived in a nursing home after becoming progressively more debilitated herself. My expression must have given me away. "I have two wonderful daughters. My husband was a very decent fellow. And I wasn't sick a day in my life until I was practically eighty. When I did get sick, the changes were pretty gradual, so I had time to adjust."

"You are a remarkable person to see things that way."

Catherine shrugged. "I inherited my disposition from my mother. Her favorite expression was 'There's no point crying over spilled milk.' She taught me to look on the bright side of things, to make do."

"It doesn't seem fair that you should have developed lymphoma on top of heart disease."

"Life isn't fair. I never expected it to be." Her tone was sharp, as though perhaps she felt life had been particularly unfair to her. Then she softened. "I was surprised by the cancer. I thought for sure my heart would give out before I had a chance to develop anything else. But really, I've been lucky there, too. Other than the time my lungs filled up with fluid, the cancer hasn't bothered me at all."

When I marveled at Catherine Endicott, it was not solely because of the way she handled her medical problems. I was impressed by her dignity in the face of adversity generally, and her ability to extend herself to others, no matter where she was. In the middle of our conversation, Catherine's roommate called out, "I can't! I can't!"

Catherine looked alarmed. "What's the matter, Ruth?"

"I can't!" her roommate repeated.

Polite as always, Catherine excused herself, used the side arms of her chair to propel herself to a standing position, took hold of her walker, and made her way to the other side of the curtain. She found her roommate struggling to put on her sweater.

"Let me help you." Ruth had her sweater upside down and was intently trying to insert her arm into the wrong sleeve. She clearly recognized Catherine and was palpably pleased to see her.

"I'm stuck," Ruth managed to say. Catherine carefully and methodically went over to the woman, who was by now hopelessly entangled in her sweater, put down her walker, gently took the sweater, and guided Ruth's arms into the sleeves.

"That's better," Catherine observed, not the least bit condescendingly. Ruth, whose social graces were preserved despite her dementia, thanked her profusely.

"Never mind that it's eighty degrees in here and I don't think she really needs a sweater," Catherine commented after she returned to her side of the double room. "She's very confused. But she did seem to want to wear that sweater."

"You're very patient," I told Catherine. "And a big help."

"At least I can do something for her." I remembered a previous roommate, who had also had dementia, whom Catherine had routinely helped into and out of bed. Eventually I realized that Catherine's episodes of angina were triggered by exertion and that her major form of exertion was assisting her roommate. With great difficulty, the staff, together with Catherine's daughters, persuaded her that she should call a nurse's aide and not do any physical maneuvering herself.

Five minutes after the sweater crisis, we were again interrupted, this time by a nursing assistant who came to escort Catherine to a podiatry appointment elsewhere in the building.

"Maria! You're back! Did you have a nice vacation?" Catherine, who knew everything about everyone who lived on her floor, also kept track of the comings and goings of the staff.

"It was very nice, thank you."

"Maria went back to Haiti to see her family," Catherine explained. Like many of the aides, Maria was from the West Indies. She was reserved, and tended to avoid eye contact. Catherine paid no attention to her seeming standoffishness. "Is your mother all right? Did she go to the doctor?"

"The doctor said there's nothing he can do. He said she has stomach cancer."

"I'm sorry to hear that. So, it's not good?"

Maria shook her head. "It's bad, very bad."

"Well, then, the best medicine was for you to visit her. Did you bring the baby?" Catherine evidently knew how many children Maria had, their ages, and their genders.

"I brought the baby. I had to pay for a seat for him on the airplane, but I took him."

Catherine looked straight at Maria, and the strength and kindness of her gaze seemed to make the young woman raise her eyes from the floor and look back. "You did a wonderful thing, Maria. I'm sure of it." She got up and the two of them went off to the podiatrist.

Whenever I asked Catherine what kept her going, what was important to her, she said it was her family. I had no doubt that her children, and to a lesser extent their spouses, their children, and, most recently, their grandchildren, were the sustaining factor in Catherine's life. Nothing gave her greater joy than seeing her family or learning of their accomplishments. Nothing made her sadder than hearing of a loss or disappointment they suffered. For Leyla Keribar, too, happiness was synonymous with being with her family. Jack Simon likewise derived tremendous satisfaction from being with his wife and from visits by his three children. Ben Frank's wife had been the sun about whom he revolved; when she died, he was lost, until gradually he learned to reestablish a connection to his daughter, a relationship that fully blossomed only in the last weeks of his life. Those frail elders who have the greatest difficulty coping are those who have no family, such as Catherine Endicott's former neighbor, who died of smoke inhalation, sick and alone.

In Catherine's case, family ties were not the only relationships that sustained her. What gave meaning to her life on a day-to-day basis were *all* her human interactions. Catherine Endicott would transform a simple request for a Tylenol into an act of redemption. Rather than feeling burdened by yet another request from another demanding patient, the nurse would feel she had the opportunity to do a good deed. Catherine praised and encouraged the nursing staff, not obsequiously but through genuine, heartfelt appreciation. Instead of confining her commentary to criticism when something was done poorly, she wrote letters to the relevant supervisors when something was done well. All the nursing assistants wanted to help care for Catherine because she had a reputation for treating everyone around her with respect and compassion. In addition to helping staff enjoy their work by bonding with them, she endeared herself to the other nursing home residents by helping them out when she could and by eschewing the gossip that sometimes poisoned the atmosphere.

Catherine Endicott was not unique: human relationships form the centerpiece of the spiritual lives of frail individuals. When friends die or move away—to live near their children or to move into an assisted-living facility or nursing home—frail people often suffer as much as from their physical disabilities. They need relationships for sustenance almost as much as they need food and shelter. Catherine Endicott was a master of the art of connecting. Without artifice or pretense, she had the capacity to reach out to those around her, with no regard for social class, race, or educational attainment. Intuitively, she grasped that far more important than fame or prestige, wealth or occupational success, are our ties to other human beings.

Leyla Keribar

The funeral for Leyla was beautiful. It took place on one of those tantalizing February days that gives the first hint that winter might not last forever. The temperature was mild—warm enough to melt the snow left over from the previous week's storm. It was the sort of weather that made the crocuses bloom prematurely and that convinced the mourners that though a life had come to an end, new life was about to emerge. Icicles shimmered, dripping steadily as the bright sun shrank them to nothingness.

The eulogy was deeply moving, capturing Leyla's many strengths and the power of her spirit. She had endured much: a troubled childhood, an oppressive political regime, physical hardship. She had suffered emotional turmoil, even when she was finally secure, living in a safe country, in her daughter's comfortable home. Leyla had always given: To her husband, she had given affection, excellent cuisine, and a lovely daughter, though perhaps not in that order. To her daughter, she had given an education, ambition, values, and her love. Her grandchildren were the most recent beneficiaries of her generosity—she had doled out advice and food as well as gifts, such as a portable television, of which Valerie did not always approve.

Friends and family came to the service. Neighbors came who had known Leyla when she lived with Valerie and George, neighbors whose children regarded Leyla as a substitute grandmother. Her bridge partners came. The other women who had worked with her on Museum of Fine Arts fund-raisers showed up. One of the other "lunch ladies" from the nearby public school who had worked with Leyla came, though she herself was eighty-five and in failing health.

"It's funny," Valerie told me over a cup of coffee months later. "The funeral helped remind me what a strong, capable woman my mother was. The last couple of years were so rough, and she was so miserable and needy, that I almost forgot."

"I guess that's what funerals are for, in part. To help solidify the memories, the good memories."

"Sometimes I think the bad memories drive out the good ones."

"We remember the incidents associated with the strongest emotions. Mildly pleasurable episodes are a lot harder to recall than the really painful ones." Research on memory demonstrates the powerful effect of emotions in facilitating the retrieval of stored information. Facts and data are not simply stashed away in the brain's analogue to a filing cabinet: they tend to be dispersed over several parts of the brain. Recalling an event is not simply a matter of opening the right file. Associated facts and feelings are key in regenerating past events.[10]

"Maybe that's why I remembered so many of the negative things in my mother's life. Fortunately, many people at the funeral had strong positive memories that they shared with everyone. My mother really was an amazing woman, you know."

When a frail person dies, as with anyone who dies after a protracted period of chronic disease rather than after a brief illness, the survivors often have to deal with contradictory emotions. On the one hand, they are saddened by the loss of a friend or relative. On the other hand, they may experience a profound sense of relief that the exquisitely slow dying process has finally come to an end. Some people may already have begun grieving for the individual who once was, perhaps months or even years earlier. The deceptively dry eyes at the funeral may be testimony to the fact that so much weeping has already taken place that families have no more tears to shed.

Much of the grieving that occurs before a frail person dies is done in private. After death comes, grief is typically more public. Every religion and culture has its own rituals to help individuals deal with the loss. Catholics hold a wake, staying with the body to show their respect. Jews sit shivah for seven days, a time during which they stay at home and friends stop over to share memories of the deceased, to bring food, and just to be together. Hindus have the ceremony known as Sreda, in which food is brought for the Brahmins and rites are performed for the dead.[11] These customs serve to provide support to the mourners and to help them remember the one they have lost. After death, only memory endures, and the survivors need stimulation and structure to preserve their memories. Trading anecdotes, looking at old pictures, talking about quirks and idiosyncrasies, all strengthen the image that would otherwise rapidly fade.

Valerie found the funeral for her mother uplifting, and the

many visitors who came to her home afterward tremendously comforting. For the first time in years, she received explicit acknowledgment of how much she had suffered in caring for her mother. For the first time in many months, she was also able to focus on the capable woman her mother had been, to see her as vibrant and active, not anxious and dependent. For two weeks, Valerie did not go to work and did not shop or clean. She let her friends bring her their elaborate home-cooked meals, commenting that the last time she had eaten so well was when her mother did the cooking.

The most difficult part of losing her mother, Valerie would discover, came later. It would start when she resumed the routine of her life, when she realized she was expected to act as though everything were perfectly normal. Valerie was reminded of her mother every day when she walked through the garden apartment her mother had once inhabited. For a time, Valerie avoided the garden apartment. She even put away the photographs of her mother she kept on her desk in order not to be reminded of her. Just when she finally went through an entire day without thinking about Leyla, a friend died, and she had another funeral to attend. Then, when Valerie felt her life truly was back to normal, Mother's Day rolled around, and she again experienced an enormous void. Valerie made a pilgrimage to the nursing home where her mother had spent the last couple of years of her life. She found it comforting to see the few remaining nursing home residents who remembered her mother, and to talk to the staff, who had been so caring. Perhaps because they had shared so much, perhaps because everyone at the nursing home was accustomed to frailty and death, perhaps because the pace was a little slower than in the outside world, Valerie felt at peace.

We resumed our conversation. Valerie told me about how Leyla and Imre had left everything behind in Turkey to start a new life in the United States when they were in their sixties. "They had to pretend they were just coming to visit. When they got here, they applied for asylum. If they had sold anything valuable, or sent packages ahead, the officials might have been suspicious. So they just abandoned everything and started over."

"Your parents must have been very courageous."

Valerie nodded and then looked puzzled. "How could someone as brave as my mother have been so terrified at the end of her life? She gave up all her friends, everything, without remorse, but then she couldn't bear to be alone in our house. And the calling out to the nurses in the nursing home—she couldn't stand being apart from other people, even for a few minutes."

"Maybe there's a connection. Maybe she was so needy because she had lost so much. Or perhaps it's that her coping skills were destroyed by her worsening dementia. Previously she had been able to handle adversity. She managed to withstand one blow after another. She dealt with the arthritis. She dealt with the Parkinson's. But at some point, it became too much. Losing her sharpness was the final straw."

Valerie resonated with the idea that the development of dementia had been a watershed in her mother's existence. "I don't think I understood what was happening at the time. Mom just seemed more anxious, more demanding, more dependent. She didn't seem radically different just because her memory began failing."

"Of course she *wasn't* radically different. Her basic personality was unchanged."

Valerie disagreed. "In some ways, of course, she was the same. She was generous. She was devoted to me. But it was as though something snapped in her brain. She was *similar* to the person she had once been, but she was also very much changed. I think that's what was so confusing."

I listened, curious to understand better. "You know, many people think of each person's life as a story, a story with chapters, but with common themes. They even talk of a kind of narrative integrity in a person's life—of wanting to be sure, for instance, that decisions about medical care are consistent with the way the person lived her life."[12]

"That's a beautiful image—life as a novel," Valerie said. "But it's not always like that. People can change. They can develop and mature, in a positive way, don't you think?"

I nodded. "I guess some people's lives are marked by radical *discontinuity*. That can be a good thing or it can be most unfortunate."

"Like with my mother."

"Like with your mother. Near the end of her life, she wasn't quite the same person she had been. So what would have made sense for her in the past—in terms of medical care, for instance—was no longer the right approach."

Valerie agreed. "My mother, who was always self-reliant and proud, became incredibly needy. And as her personality changed, my view of what kind of medical treatment she would want changed, too. Mom had always loved life; she loved people and culture. She couldn't stand staying home. When my father was ill, she didn't like being with him for long stretches—she felt she had to go downtown, to a museum, to a meeting. She drove me and George crazy with her restlessness. Especially since I ended up having to take care of my father. I just couldn't understand her priorities. But I think she had such zest for life—and for so many years had lived in such a restrictive society—that she felt driven, she felt she had to be on the go. Once she lost her animation, I didn't think she wanted to live anymore. Before the dementia, I'm sure she would have wanted any treatment that could help keep her alive. Afterward, everything was totally different."

The waitress came by and refilled our coffee cups. For a few moments, we focused on the coffee, on adding just the right amount of cream and sugar.

I took a few sips and decided to ask Valerie what I knew would be a painful question. "Do you think your mother found meaning in her life, despite all her problems?"

Valerie hesitated. "As long as she was engaged with other people, I think she felt her life was meaningful. When she lived with us and the boys were at home, she was a second mother to them. Better than a mother, because she accepted them uncritically. They loved her. And they loved her cooking. She was a great cook."

"But your sons have been grown up for some time."

"Well, maybe not grown up, but out of the house, off to college," Valerie corrected me. "But then Mother had her work at the school. She wasn't just a lunch lady. She learned all the children's names in the elementary school. She noticed if they were sad and called them over to talk to her after lunch. She noticed if there was a child who didn't like the main course and made sure he got two portions of French fries or two desserts to tide him over."

"She was still gracious and generous until the very end," I observed.

"But she turned inward. Everything was me, me, me."

"She was self-absorbed. She couldn't reach out the way she once had. But I remember a time, not that long before she died, when one of the nurses implored your mother to stop crying out because she, the nurse, had a migraine. And your mother, preoccupied with herself as she was, pulled herself together and managed to give that nurse a little peace. She really rose to the challenge."

Valerie was very moved. She was impressed that the nursing home staff had seen beyond the demanding, dependent person her mother had become to the kind, compassionate person she had always been.

"There was another time I remember when your mother amazed us all. One of the nursing assistants had a death in the family. A baby—a premature baby. Leyla always asked about the aides' families. When she heard about the preemie, she was so distraught that she forget her own woes." I waited to let that sink in. "At the memorial service for your mother at the nursing home, that nursing assistant spoke out about how touched she had been by Leyla's thoughtfulness."

"I remember that, now that you mention it."

"The aide just wished there had been more moments like that, when your mother could reach out to others. Without that connectedness, she did not have a sense of purpose."

"I don't think she found life meaningful anymore. Her losses were too great. She couldn't interact with others in a way that made her feel useful. And I think that terrifying childhood memories came back to haunt her. Maybe she would have been better able to deal with her situation if she had been a religious person. Unfortunately, she was always resolutely secular."

"You did the only thing you could, Valerie. You tried to help her overcome the free-floating anxiety, the helplessness, that destroyed her zest for life. When you found you could not make her comfortable emotionally, you sought to keep her physically comfortable. When she developed pneumonia, we brought her fever down and eased her breathing. She's at peace now." We drained our coffee cups.

Religious faith might have helped Lelya Keribar during a period of profound spiritual malaise, as it helped Will Merlin, Ben Frank's bench friend, during a period of physical distress. Many religious traditions view human beings as the instruments of

God's will. From this perspective, life has meaning because people are part of a divine plan, however opaque that plan may be to mere mortals. Religion imbues existence with significance because it typically locates a divine spark within every person, regardless of that individual's "contribution" to society. Partaking of holiness is a way to experience life as meaningful. A belief in an afterlife likewise transforms the drive to find meaning in everyday existence: if life on earth is just a brief moment in an eternity of being, then the pressure to achieve or to produce or to succeed in the here and now diminishes.

Membership in a well-defined cultural group with its own traditions and rituals can similarly give frail older people a global sense of purpose. Some cultures, such as traditional Chinese society, value their oldest members highly, believing them to be sources of wisdom. Not only is care of the frail elderly an assumed responsibility of the children, but the elderly maintain a sense of worth by virtue of retaining a role within the family structure. Multigenerational households are conducive to frail individuals' participating in family life and feeling important. The communitarian life on an Israeli kibbutz is another way of incorporating the older person with significant disabilities into daily life and finding tasks that she can perform. In a society in which everyone engages in menial chores and shares in responsibility for the welfare of the whole, it is easier to come up with genuinely useful jobs for their frailest members.

Jack Simon

If there was one fixed point in Jack Simon's life, one rock of stability, it was his wife, Peggy. She had made it possible for him to come home after his stroke, she had reassured him when he was beset by anxiety in the face of failing vision due to his cataract. Jack had always made a point of planning for the future: he had faced the prospect of illness and ultimately death by choosing a health-care proxy and by completing a will. He had never planned for the possibility of life without Peggy. When she unexpectedly died, suffering from a massive heart attack, he was devastated.

"I never imagined I would outlive her. Never!" he told me when I went to see him on my nursing home rounds at Park Village. He was no longer living in his own apartment—almost immediately after Peggy died, he discovered that he could not take care of himself. He moved into the nursing home on the grounds of the Village, the backup facility that had been one of the reasons for selecting the continuing-care retirement community in the first place.[13] "I miss her terribly," he added.

"You'd been married for a long time."

"Sixty years. Can you believe that?"

"Not too many people stay together for sixty years these days. It must be very hard to wake up in the morning and realize she's not there next to you." Jack was too choked up to answer. "Obviously you're very sad. But are you managing? Are you eating your meals? Are you sleeping at night?"

Jack nodded. "My kids keep me going. Mark lives out of state, but he telephones every week. Ginny and Stuart have their own busy lives, but one visits on Saturday and one on Sunday. And the grandchildren come when they can. I'm a great-grandfather now, you know," he added. He wheeled himself over to his bureau, rummaged in the top drawer, and produced a small photo of a beaming baby. "That's the most recent addition. Just six months old." I made the expected noises about how handsome the baby was.

There was nothing wrong with Jack Simon's memory. He

could rattle off the names and ages of his three children, his five grandchildren, and his two great-grandchildren. I asked him if the whole family ever got together.

"They're coming for my eighty-fourth birthday. It's next month, you know. It was supposed to be a surprise party, but Ginny figured they better ask my permission. I wasn't sure they should go ahead with it, but we decided it would be a good way to get the whole family together. We're renting a private dining room in a hotel. My brother and sister are coming, too—one sister passed away, so it's just the three of us left. I expect we'll be about thirty people altogether."

I wished Jack a happy birthday and then moved on to inquire about his physical state. "How's the walking?"

"Not good. I got an electric wheelchair so I can get around better. I do pretty well with my buddy here," he said, slapping the wheels of his chair affectionately. "It bothered me at first, but now I don't really mind. I'm tired a lot, though. I doze off every afternoon and don't seem to have the energy I used to have."

I decided to check Jack's blood for anemia or an underactive thyroid gland, either of which could contribute to his fatigue. We also discussed the possibility of the spread of his prostate cancer, which had been quiescent for two years, and agreed to measure the PSA as well. All the tests proved normal.

"I guess I'm just getting old," Jack concluded on my next scheduled visit to the nursing home, thirty days later.

The next few months were difficult. Jack was moody. He was often very sad. I asked him how he spent his time to determine if he was depressed or just appropriately sad.

Jack immediately brightened up. "I've taken over as president of the Men's Club. There aren't too many men around here—three-quarters of the residents are women. And half the men don't have all their marbles. The few who are left like to get together every week. Sometimes we have a speaker and then a discussion. Sometimes I pick out an article from the newspaper to talk about. And every month we go out to a restaurant."

I could see that the Men's Club was a continuation of Jack's previous work coaching middle-aged executives who had lost their jobs. The earlier activity had been a mixture of the therapeutic and the practical; the current activity was a combination of the therapeutic and the social, with some intellectual stimulation thrown in. The very fact that this group of men could use their minds gave them tremendous satisfaction, quite apart from what they actually discussed.

"I'm also on the Residents' Council," Jack continued. The council was composed of patient representatives from each wing of the nursing home. They met twice a month to discuss issues bearing on their quality of life, whether it was planning a breakfast buffet to accommodate early and late risers or coming up with a satisfactory list of outings.

Fascinating work on "learned helplessness" demonstrated that nursing home residents who remain in control of some aspects of their lives stay healthier than those who have everything done for them.[14] In addition, surveys of nursing home residents asking what was important to them revealed that issues directly affecting their quality of life—such as what they ate and how gently they were treated—were of greater concern to them than their medical or nursing care.[15] Jack had automatically gravitated toward those facets of nursing home life that were likely to enhance the meaning of his life.

"We set up a Menu Committee at the last Residents' Council meeting. I'm chairing it. We're meeting with the new director of food services and the new chef to see if we can have more variety in the meals. They have a rotation system, you know. It's a ten-day cycle. Different choices every day for ten days and then it starts all over again. Though that's misleading—the backup option if you don't like the main selection only changes a couple of times a week."

I commented that the food could not be too bad, since Jack had gained five pounds in the preceding three months.

"Too many snacks," Jack confessed. "But if the meals were better, I wouldn't be so hungry for an evening snack. Also, they serve dinner at five o'clock. Half the residents are in bed by seven." Jack shook his head. "Generally they treat us like three-year-olds. If you don't go to bed at seven, and you eat supper at five, you're ready for a little something by ten. Also, it's a long stretch until breakfast."

I marveled at Jack's energy, despite his complaints of fatiguing easily. He seemed to have found a niche in the nursing home, as a sort of activist/community organizer. I wondered how long his activities in the Men's Club, on the Residents' Council, and on the Menu Committee would be sufficient to give him a sense of fulfillment.

On a subsequent visit to the nursing home several months later, I started with my usual open-ended question: "So, how are things?"

"Pretty good," Jack answered cagily. I inquired about his arthritis and whether he was having any difficulty urinating. We reviewed the status of his vision and his mobility. I was putting my stethoscope away in anticipation of leaving when Jack stopped me cold. "I have a question for you. I heard on television that it was normal for men to be interested in women—at any age. But for someone in my condition, is it safe?"

I assured him that older men were no more immune to sexually transmitted diseases than younger men were, but that otherwise sex was safe. A significant fraction of older men had problems with erectile function, however. "Is this a theoretical question or," I stumbled, "a burning issue?"

Jack smiled coyly. "As a matter of fact, I have a lady friend. I've known her for a while, but I never thought of her in, well, a romantic way. She lives here, too, and she has all kinds of medical problems. But she's very sweet, and one day on impulse I just took her hand and that's how it's been ever since."

I reiterated that sexual relationships were perfectly normal among consenting adults, regardless of age. "At least you don't have to worry about your friend becoming pregnant," I added. I was a bit concerned that Jack might discover he had the interest but not the ability. He did not have high blood pressure, the condition most commonly associated with impotence, but he had had a stroke, so he had some degree of vascular disease. Among his medications, the hormone treatment for prostate cancer had the potential to produce impotence. I mentioned this possibility and then emphasized that there were many ways of expressing both amorous and sexual feelings.

When I went to the nurses' station to write my monthly progress note, I was dismayed to find that the staff was in a tizzy over Jack's behavior toward his friend Cheryl. The other residents called him a dirty old man for holding hands in the communal living room. One nurse wanted to know if I could prescribe a pill to curb his "hypersexuality." The nursing home social worker had already been called in to "protect" Cheryl. I was stunned and indignant. I had just finished preparing Jack for the possibility that he would be physically unable to have sexual intercourse, but it had not occurred to me that he might be socially unable.

Sexuality in the elderly in general and in the nursing home in particular remains a taboo subject. Despite growing theoreti-

cal knowledge of sexual function in the elderly, actual acceptance of sexual relationships is often halfhearted at best. When
Viagra was introduced in 1998 as a treatment for impotence,
the assumption was that it was a drug for middle-aged men
rather than for older men. Elderly men might be impotent,
but whether they were was thought to be of little consequence
since surely they were not interested in sex. Or if they were
interested, no self-respecting woman would be interested in a
man who was seventy-five or eighty-five, so potency was
thought to be unimportant. In fact, an estimated two-thirds
of men aged seventy are impotent, and they are apt to be distressed by the problem.[16] Physical factors are commonly the
basis for erectile dysfunction, principally diabetes, heart disease, and medications.[17]

In the nursing home, expressions of sexuality are difficult
because of the attitudes of staff and other residents, because of
the lack of privacy, and occasionally because of institutional
policies. Views of what constitutes appropriate behavior often
interfere with the ability of nursing home residents to have a
sexual relationship. Because the nursing home is a closed environment—some would argue that it is a "total institution,"
like a mental asylum—the community necessarily sets standards for acceptable conduct. Activities that would be eminently reasonable in another milieu, including public displays
of affection, may, in fact, be rejected by the majority of nursing home residents. Balancing the autonomy of the individual
against collective rights is not always easy. Ideally, both the
couple and the community will be satisfied by using a private
room for all but the most modest amorous demonstrations.

Enabling nursing home residents to relate sexually is particularly problematic if one or both members of the couple
have some degree of cognitive impairment. The desire of staff

to protect their charges against predators, particularly predatory men, is dramatic when the man is intact and the woman has mild to moderate dementia. Surely, the staff argues, the woman is being taken advantage of and cannot truly consent to overtures by an "aggressive" male. In fact, demented individuals retain primitive drives such as the sexual urge. A resident who can no longer read a newspaper or write a letter or find her way to the dining room may be quite capable of figuring out what the man sitting next to her means when he puts his arm around her. She can no longer feel a thrill of mastery from solving a difficult problem, but she may be perfectly able to delight in the affection of another human being.

Not only do nurses and social workers often bring their own prejudices about what is an appropriate relationship to the nursing home setting, but so do family members.[18] For a devoted daughter to see her father caressing a woman other than her mother, even if her mother has been dead for several years, can be difficult. She may insist that the nursing home "break up" the relationship. In fact, the daughter might have been equally skeptical of her father's earlier choice of partner, before he moved into the nursing home, but she was not in a position to do anything about it. Once her father was institutionalized, she began to see herself as his protector and advocate. She became accustomed to serving as his voice in the nursing home, requesting a change in diet on his behalf, or complaining that he wore dirty and wrinkled clothing, or pleading with his physician to discontinue the anti-anxiety medications, which she believed were making him sleepy and confused. Seeking to extricate him from what she regarded as a destructive relationship came naturally to her. When faced with an insistent family member's demands that her father be prevented from seeing another resident, the nursing home staff finds it difficult to counter that his "autonomy" requires that he be able to socialize with whomever he chooses.

Jack and Cheryl were among the few lucky couples who were both cognitively intact and also had supportive families. Cheryl's daughter Kelly lived in the area and invited both Jack and Cheryl to her home for Thanksgiving dinner. Jack's son Stuart, who had no family of his own, flew up to join them and help maneuver his father and his wheelchair.

Jack and Cheryl found the dinner almost as exhausting as their hostess did. They were no longer accustomed to so much commotion. Jack was embarrassed that he needed his son to help him use the bathroom, since it was not equipped with a raised toilet seat or grab bars, unlike the bathroom in the nursing home. He was afraid his wheelchair would leave tire marks on Kelly's beautiful hardwood floors. He was afraid that Kelly and the other relatives would not approve of him. His long dormant sense of insecurity about his lack of education suddenly made him tongue-tied. Being dependent on his son for a ride home made him even more nervous: he felt he could not simply decide to leave if the anxiety became overwhelming.

When they finally returned to the nursing home, both Jack and Cheryl were tremendously relieved. Despite Jack's fears, nothing untoward had occurred. Kelly actually seemed to approve of her mother's choice of male companion. She had even muttered that he was much more of a gentleman than her own father had been. Jack gave Cheryl a quick kiss before heading to his own room for the night.

Jack Simon's relationships with women—first with his wife and later with a lady friend—and his participation in a variety of activities at Park Village were possible because of his positive attitude and his determination.[19] His ability to transcend his deficits and remain fully engaged with life was also possible because of technology. Perhaps the most liberating assistive device was his electric wheelchair. A conventional wheelchair increased his mobility, but his right arm, weak from his stroke, did not permit him to travel far. He could not negotiate inclines. The best he could do with the standard chair was to go short distances on level ground, or else he needed a person to push him. The electric wheelchair dramatically expanded the territory he could cover. Jack could get from one end of the continuing-care retirement community to the other on his own: he could reach the auditorium for concerts, the main dining room for meals, the on-site library, and the exercise room. His freedom greatly enhanced, he found ways to give to the surrounding community.

Shortly after his stroke, Jack's executive advisees had given him speech-recognition software as a present. The product they gave him was fairly primitive, requiring that he pause between words. He found it awkward and unnatural to use. Two years later, speech-recognition technology took a great leap forward—it became possible to dictate using continuous speech. Jack had to buy a computer with a faster processor and more memory, but then, after a ten-minute training session, he could speak directly into a microphone and his words would appear on the screen instantly. He had to articulate clearly and consistently, sometimes selecting from a menu of possible interpretations of his words when the computer was uncertain about what he said. With a little practice and a few helpful tips from the customer-support service, Jack found he could write much faster than he had ever been able to by hand or by typing. He could send letters, he could prepare notes to use when he lectured his students (the unemployed executives he periodically coached), and he discovered email. With email he could communicate with his children even if he did not have a great deal to report. Somehow, sending email when he had just a couple of sentences to write made sense, though writing only a few words on a piece of embossed stationery did not. Jack would never have dictated personal letters to another person to transcribe, and he would never have hired a secretary to record his lecture notes. Without his speech-recognition system, Jack would quite simply have been cut off from what proved to be two major sources of satisfaction in his life.

Some of the technology on which Jack Simon relied was very simple—no electronics, no microchips, and, in some instances, no electricity. He used a special shoehorn with a long handle that allowed him to put on his own shoes—a feat he would have been unable to perform if he had needed to bend down. He had a special telephone with large, clearly labeled buttons so that he could place calls despite limited dexterity. His clothing was tailored to the needs of a man who had trouble handling zippers and buttons: he wore sweat pants with elastic waists and slip-on shoes without laces. He switched from a conventional razor to an electric shaver. These simple interventions diminished Jack's dependence on other people and enhanced his autonomy: he needed help showering in the morning, but for the remainder of the day, he was fairly independent. He could lie down and take a nap whenever he pleased, as long as he could transfer from his chair to his bed and kick off his shoes. He could go to a lecture, knowing that if he wanted to leave in the middle, he would not have to wait for an attendant to escort him.

What is striking about all four of the people whose stories I tell in this book is that they did not *feel* old. They did not think of themselves as any different from their younger, more vigorous selves.[20] Their sense of identity was essentially unchanged, even as their bodies and minds became unreliable. Since their personalities were fundamentally preserved, and their styles of coping with life's vicissitudes were unchanged, their means of deriving satisfaction from existence were, not surprisingly, consistent with earlier patterns. The activities and approaches that gave meaning to their lives were of a piece with previous activities. Catherine Endicott did not become compassionate all of a sudden: she exhibited her sensitivity to others in new ways and new settings, but basically the nature of her relationships was maintained. Jack Simon's work with his wife promoting literacy was a variant on his earlier career as an adviser to executives who had lost their jobs.

Finding meaning despite frailty proves easier than predicted, despite the losses of work and status that often come with old age, because meaning so often depends on emotional involvement with other people. For Ben Frank, Jack Simon, Catherine Endicott, and Leyla Keribar, being with family was probably their single most meaningful pastime. Friendships—both new and old—can be another source of meaning. Ben Frank made a friend while sitting on a bench in his neighborhood. Though their relationship was only of brief duration, the connectedness Ben experienced was as uplifting as a potent antidepressant. Catherine Endicott renewed old friendships at the assisted-living facility, where she was reunited with women from the neighborhood of her youth. Conversely, the loss of friendships can be devastating, as when Margaret Simon's closest friend died, reducing her entire world to that of her frail husband. And the lack of a sense of meaning in life arose most commonly when emotional and cognitive problems impaired the capacity to establish and maintain relationships, as with Leyla Keribar.

To have a sense of purpose, frail older people need to possess a certain measure of autonomy. They need to be able to make choices. Jack Simon's decision to undergo hormonal treatment for prostate cancer gave him enough of a sense of control over his own life that he was able to embark on a project with his wife to intervene in the lives of others. Catherine Endicott's decision to work as a volunteer in the local library gave her a goal to strive for, as well as structure to her life and something to do. Older people do not have to be fully independent in *implementing* their decisions—they may need help in getting to the library or in reading information for the cancer support group. But hearing, seeing, walking, and other basic functions are tremendously helpful in *facilitating* autonomy. Fixing Jack's cataract, getting Ben a hearing aid, and replacing Leyla's hip had a major impact on their ability to pursue meaningful activities.

Deriving satisfaction from life requires *action* as well as autonomy. A merely passive existence is seldom sufficient: doing, creating, initiating, seem to be essential, however small the scale. Baking, playing the piano, knitting, teaching, and praying are all activities that can play a spiritual role for frail older individuals. Ben Frank's friend Will relied on prayer; Leyla Keribar achieved a sense of peace from playing the piano. One of the major reasons why depression is so devastating, particularly to frail older people, is because the apathy and indifference it engenders turn people from activity to passivity. For someone such as Ben Frank, whose quiet personality and physical weakness conspired to render him passive, the addition of depressive symptoms to the mix had profoundly negative consequences.

Older people also need to feel part of something larger than themselves. One of the quintessential features of being human is the awareness and fear of mortality, and those who are frail are exquisitely conscious of the imminence of death.[21] People need "immortality projects" to sustain themselves in the face of their earthly transience. Such projects can include writing books, or designing products, or simply passing along one's genes through children and grandchildren. Older individuals can achieve this sense of immortality identification with a cultural or religious tradition. Perceiving themselves as linked to the past allows them to feel part of a human chain, implicitly linked to the future as well. The sense of being part of something larger than oneself was the motivation for Jack Simon to participate in support groups for men with prostate cancer and to join the Residents' Council. Instead of remaining an isolated individual residing in the nursing home, he chose to band together with others to introduce change to the facility and to strive to improve the quality of life for all the residents.

Old age often brings with it a tension between ego integrity and despair.[22] For those whose old age is marked by frailty, the pull toward despair is sometimes very powerful. As a counterweight, however, the frail older person has had eighty years or more in which to establish his or her sense of identity. That sense of self, along with a sense of values and purpose, is not so readily undermined by a handful of physical ailments. People do not think of themselves as *old* just because they have their eightieth birthday. Rather, they deal with problems and disability when they arise, just as they always have.[23] Moreover, meaning is not necessarily acquired from a single concrete accomplishment; instead it derives from the many smaller activities that constitute a person's daily routine. It was those little acts of caring that kept Catherine Endicott going, those moments of reaching out to others that sustained Ben Frank and Jack Simon, and the contacts with family that mattered to them all.

CHAPTER 6

Facing Frailty: Prevention and Social Responsibility

The theme of this book is that frailty is a part of contemporary life. The price for the longevity that we gained in the second half of the twentieth century is a period of frailty before death for an increasingly large number of people. While the rate of frailty varies depending on the precise definition chosen, 22 percent of women and 15 percent of men over age sixty-five either reside in a nursing home or need help in order to stay out of a nursing home. These rates triple after the age of eighty-five.[1] The challenge to those of us who are frail and to the families of the frail is to come to terms with frailty, to learn to value those who are frail, and to help them value themselves. In addition, the challenge to those of us who are not frail is to try to avoid becoming frail, and the challenge to the society as a whole is to design better environments to support the frail elderly and to create systems of medical care that promote both autonomy and comfort.

Prevention

Ben Frank, Catherine Endicott, Jack Simon, and Leyla Keribar were already well on the road to frailty when they first made their appearance in this book: preventive strategies could probably have done little to alter their course. Moreover, their frailty was largely unavoidable—the Parkinson's disease and osteoarthritis that made Leyla Keribar frail and the stroke that rendered Jack Simon frail could not have been prevented. But even if frailty is not a condition against which we can reliably immunize ourselves with a pill or a shot, there are measures that can help prevent this troubling condition. Prevention of frailty is a goal to which we can all aspire—young and old, physicians and patients, individuals and society as a whole. The dream of geriatric medicine is to shrink the period of severe disability before death to a minimum. In the idealized vision of the life cycle, people would remain vigorous into their eighties or nineties, possibly even past one hundred, and then abruptly succumb to a single, decisive, acute illness. Such a trajectory would eliminate frailty altogether: the transition between robust health and death would last days or, at most, weeks. Instead of a protracted period during which one organ after another goes into decline—the heart, the kidneys, the brain—translating into marked diminution of function for the person whose organs are failing, we would witness the sudden collapse of one or more critical systems, followed rapidly by death.

Preventive strategies *do* exist, but they must be advocated sensitively and realistically, acknowledging their powerful potential but also their lamentable limitations. The interventions that deserve particular attention are those for which there is compelling evidence of efficacy—interventions that stand a chance of having a major impact on frailty. Since frailty arises from the interaction of factors in multiple domains—emotional, physical, cognitive, and social—the best strategy for preventing or postponing frailty is to target the leading problems that arise in each of these spheres. In the psychological arena, one critical problem warranting treatment is depression; in the physical realm, exercise is among the most important interventions; in the cognitive arena, a useful strategy is treatment of high blood pressure; and in the social domain, social networks of family and friends are tremendously helpful.

In the *psychological arena*, depression is the single most common psychiatric problem afflicting the elderly, and one with potentially devastating consequences. At least 15 percent of elderly people who live in their own homes have frequent, oppressive symptoms of sadness or worthlessness of sufficient magnitude to interfere with their daily lives, though a much smaller percentage has the full-blown psychiatric syndrome known as depression. In the hospital, as many as 10 percent of elderly patients have depression, and in the nursing home, the rate is higher still: as many as 15 percent of residents are depressed.[2] Depression can be difficult to diagnose in the elderly. Some patients manifest the same symptoms as younger depressed people: they feel sad, helpless, and apathetic, and have a low sense of self-esteem. More commonly, however, older individuals have primarily physical rather than emotional symptoms: they feel tired and weak, they have trouble sleeping, and their appetite is poor. These symptoms can easily be mistaken for a physical rather than a psychological problem.

The mainstay of treatment for depression is medication. There are now several different types of highly effective drugs available. The medications that have been around longest are the tricyclic antidepressants, including amitriptyline (Elavil), nortriptyline (Pamelor), and desipramine (Norpramin). The problem with these drugs is that they tend to make people sleepy, to make them feel dizzy, to cause difficulty urinating, and to lead to falls. A chemically distinct type of medication, the selective serotonin reuptake inhibitors (SSRIs) such as fluoxetine (Prozac), sertraline (Zoloft), and paroxetine (Paxil), are increasingly popular choices for treatment of depression in the elderly. While these drugs are relatively free of side effects, they may cause gastrointestinal upset or loss of appetite. Depression is a chronic disease, and the chance of developing a recurrence is sufficiently high that current recommendations are to continue treatment for at least a year and possibly indefinitely.[3] Early diagnosis is imperative to prevent symptoms such as excessive sleepiness and poor appetite from exacerbating other physical problems and triggering frailty.

In the *physical realm,* mobility is critical to avoiding frailty, and exercise can be a potent force in maintaining mobility. It also has the virtue of being cheap and associated with only minimal risk. Not all exercises are equivalent in their effects. While aerobic exercise—exercise that increases heart rate and respiratory rate—is beneficial in maintaining or improving cardiovascular health, resistance training—activity that stimulates muscle growth—affects strength. Still other forms of exercise are designed to improve balance. Aerobic exercise has an indirect effect on frailty, primarily by helping to prevent heart attacks, which can contribute to frailty.[4] Resistance training, by contrast, works directly on mobility. This kind of exercise does not require a gym or swimming pool or even a safe place to walk: strength training of the lower extremities can be as simple as doing straight leg raising with progressively heavier weights. Gait and balance training take a variety of forms, including the traditional Chinese Tai Chi Chuan.

One of the principal ways that exercise programs can affect frailty is by the prevention of falls, which are a huge problem in the elderly.[5] Exercise can also help prevent frailty by maintaining independence in those activities necessary to remain on one's own: lifting and reaching, carrying bundles, walking down the supermarket aisles. Fortunately, it is never too late to start exercising. While it is desirable to develop a habit of regular exercise at an early age and maintain that pattern throughout life, taking up exercise in adulthood (including older adulthood) has beneficial effects.[6] Even ninety-year-old nursing home residents can increase their muscle mass through strength training, which translates into a steadier and brisker gait.[7]

In the *cognitive arena*, it is evident that a clear mind goes a long way to preventing frailty. Remaining independent despite multiple physical problems is difficult enough; in the presence of dementia, it is typically impossible. *Dementia* is a catchall term for a variety of disorders that produce a progressive loss of cognitive function in domains such as memory, judgment, and language. While Alzheimer's disease is by far the most common type of dementia and cannot as yet be prevented, vascular dementia is the second most common type of dementia, and it *may* be preventable.[8] In vascular dementia, multiple small strokes collectively produce cognitive impairment. Each individual stroke may be so small as to be imperceptible when it occurs—it does not have to result in obvious symptoms such as paralysis or the inability to speak. It can be far more subtle or, in fact, picked up only either on CAT scan or on the even more sensitive magnetic resonance imaging (MRI) scan. The cumulative effect of loss of brain tissue in many regions is dementia.

Vascular dementia is almost always due to high blood pressure. Sustained high blood pressure causes atherosclerosis, which results in the blockage of blood vessels, or stroke. There is good reason to believe that treatment of hypertension can prevent vascular dementia. A European study found that patients with high blood pressure who were treated had a 50 percent reduction in the risk of dementia compared to those who were not.[9] The good news is that we know how to treat high blood pressure and have many excellent drugs from among which to choose. However, we do not know just how far to lower blood pressure or whether there is an age beyond which blood-pressure reduction ceases to be desirable. In general, keeping systolic blood pressure below 160—the cutoff for reducing the risk of stroke—seems advisable, even in extreme old age.

Prevention of vascular dementia may have the unexpected side effect of ameliorating Alzheimer's disease as well. In a fascinating study, women from an order of nuns agreed to have their mental function studied during life and their brains studied after death. It turned out that women with the same degree of Alzheimer's changes in their brains often had very different degrees of dementia during life, apparently depending on whether there were vascular changes as well. The Alzheimer's abnormalities and the vascular changes were not simply additive: vascular changes seemed to dramatically worsen the effects of the Alzheimer's changes. Conversely, at least one nun with fairly severe Alzheimer's changes but no vascular abnormalities was cognitively intact during life. Protecting the brain against vascular dementia may have a beneficial effect in moderating the development of Alzheimer's—and in preventing frailty.[10]

In the *social domain*, the involvement of friends and family is such a powerful force in the life of the elderly that it can affect mortality. The presence of social supports is associated with an increased chance of survival after a heart attack, even taking into consideration the severity of the heart attack and the existence of other medical conditions that might be expected to influence the outcome.[11] In a chronic condition such as renal failure, in which the patient undergoes dialysis three times a week, social support also influences survival: those with a network of friends and relatives live longer than those who are more isolated.[12] Social support has a similar role in affecting the development of frailty. An old person who falls and breaks a hip is much more apt to recover without developing disability if she maintains significant contact with friends and relatives. Likewise, when an elderly person has a stroke, the major factor determining whether he will develop permanent disability is social support.[13]

No one fully understands how social connections produce beneficial effects. Conceivably, the same characteristics that promote friendships also induce physical resiliency. If social networks do act directly to avoid frailty, the implications for prevention will still be murky. People cannot be compelled to make friends. They have no control over how many cousins or siblings they have. Nonetheless, the desirability of living in close proximity to friends may be a persuasive argument against moving away from established connections to a retirement community. Alternatively, for someone who makes friends easily and whose neighbors have died or themselves moved elsewhere, a retirement community may serve as a means of establishing a new network. In our highly mobile society, where children and grandchildren often live far away from their aging relatives, and where Grandpa is often uprooted to be near family members only when he is so frail as to need a nursing home, it may make more sense for him to move nearby while he is younger and more robust. He then has the chance to develop a new social network including but not limited to his family.

Just as treating depression, maintaining mobility, treating hypertension, and promoting social supports can help counteract the tendency to become frail, so, too, can *retarding the aging process* postpone frailty. The problem with seeking to delay aging is that we do not understand what causes aging, let alone how to slow it down. The one well-documented means of experimentally extending longevity is through caloric restriction. What this means is reducing intake to near starvation levels, while maintaining a diet adequate in protein, vitamins, and minerals so as to avoid diseases of malnutrition. Prolonged periods of caloric restriction can double longevity. The catch is that the only species in which this strategy has been proved to work are rodents and insects.[14] The effect of severe caloric restriction in nonhuman primates is under investigation, but the results will not be known for decades.

One theory about the cause of aging is that it is due to oxidative damage. In the normal run of affairs, the theory goes, various cellular ingredients combine with oxygen, forming highly reactive substances called free radicals. Free radicals damage DNA, the basic genetic material. As more and more damage accumulates, deterioration of the cell develops, resulting in aging. If this theory is correct, then aging should be delayed by antioxidants, which work by neutralizing free radicals, preventing them from harming DNA.[15] One of the most promising of the antioxidants is vitamin E, a naturally occurring chemical with relatively few side effects. Researchers have found that vitamin E may slow the progression of Alzheimer's disease[16] and protects against heart disease.[17] Whether it will prove to slow aging is unknown, but many older people take vitamin E, many physicians recommend it to their patients, and quite a few geriatricians and neurologists take it themselves.

Another candidate for an antiaging tonic, at least in women, is estrogen. Estrogen has been reported to improve memory, to stave off heart disease, and to prevent osteoporotic fractures. It is decidedly beneficial in preventing osteoporosis in postmenopausal women.[18] It probably plays a role in preventing heart disease: estrogen-replacement therapy produces elevations in high density lipoprotein (HDL), the "good" cholesterol that is associated with a lower risk of heart attacks. Not all studies have demonstrated lower heart attack rates in postmenopausal women taking estrogen than in their counterparts who are not on estrogen, but the preponderance of the evidence favors a beneficial effect.[19] The effect of estrogen on memory is less clear. Healthy women are more likely to be on estrogen replacement than are otherwise comparable women who have Alzheimer's disease. Sophisticated studies of brain activity during various intellectual activities suggest that estrogen enables the brain to work better.[20] On the other hand, several carefully controlled studies have failed to show that estrogen plays any role at all in cognitive function.[21] On balance, estrogen is a desirable medication for most older women, particularly those who have had a hysterectomy and who are at low risk of breast cancer, since its main drawbacks are an increased risk of uterine and breast cancer. As modified versions of estrogen are designed that act like estrogen in the bones but not in the reproductive organs, these drugs may prove to be modest antiaging tonics for women.[22]

Many other drugs and behaviors have been advocated to prevent frailty. Some are beneficial or will turn out, after further study, to be helpful. However, most are, at best, of modest utility. They may warrant adoption in selected individuals, especially if they are cheap and devoid of side effects. Expensive remedies that are often accompanied by serious adverse reactions are best avoided.[23]

Good genes, good luck, good medical care, and a healthy dose of prevention have made the dream of a vigorous old age a reality for millions of older people today. For millions of others, frailty remains their fate. Discussions of prevention must acknowledge the prevalence of frailty, both today and for the foreseeable future, and not castigate the frail for their dependence. Blaming the victim is an all too common temptation in an environment that encourages individual responsibility for health. If we exhort people to take matters into their hands—abandoning smoking, engaging in exercise, limiting alcohol—as well we should, we must not delude ourselves that these behaviors will eradicate frailty. The danger of drawing such an extreme conclusion is that we will fail to develop systems to support those who do become frail. If we erroneously believe that frailty is on the verge of extinction, then we have no need to design better nursing homes and new alternatives to institutional care, or to promote technological innovations that enable the elderly to compensate for their deficits. If we persuade ourselves that we will never become frail, provided we take the appropriate preventive measures, then we will make inadequate financial provisions for our old age and we will not bother with advance medical planning (drawing up a living will and designating a health-care proxy). If American society does not take seriously the anticipated surge in frailty as the baby boomers reach their eighties, then we will not revamp Medicare to include coverage for long-term care.

Perhaps even more devastating than the social and economic consequences of blaming the victim are the emotional consequences. Coping with frailty is extraordinarily difficult. The four people in this book were, by and large, successful in confronting frailty, and they were blessed with personal, financial, and familial resources. None of them found their journey through frailty easy, and all of them experienced significant challenges along the way. To be held *responsible* for a condition you never wanted and that you sought to avoid can only add to the pain of frailty.

The quest for effective prevention reveals much about American culture. Ours is an individualistic society, and we would like to believe that we have a great deal of control over our lives. We want to feel that our behavior matters. In the arena of dependence and disability in old age, the complex and heterogeneous condition known as frailty, behavior does matter. Our actions can prevent frailty—to some extent. But we must also acknowledge that frailty is neither inevitable nor entirely avoidable. We must simultaneously preach prevention, concentrating our energies on those areas of greatest efficacy, and prepare ourselves to face frailty with acceptance, creativity, and compassion.

Social Strategies for Coping with Frailty

I have argued that facing frailty entails fixing the fixable part (modifying or correcting failing vision, poor hearing, or worn-out joints), ensuring access to living situations that are conducive to both autonomy and social interactions, making reasonable decisions regarding the *extent* and *type* of treatment for acute illness, and seeking meaning in life—finding satisfaction despite debility and decline.

Accepting and coping with frailty is partly the task of each frail individual, but transcending frailty is also dependent on the social context. The surrounding society can make an enormous difference to the frail by guaranteeing medical care for the conditions that plague them, such as cataracts and osteoarthritis. Ensuring care translates into paying for ancillary devices such as glasses and hearing aids, providing insurance coverage for prescription drugs that improve health and physical functioning, and making certain there is no waiting period for elective surgery. Currently, Medicare, the principal insurer for the elderly, does not pay for glasses, hearing aids, or prescription drugs. Health-maintenance organizations (HMOs) for seniors do cover glasses and have been under pressure to provide a prescription-drug benefit, which is a major bone of contention, given the rapidly rising costs facing HMOs. Surgery is readily available in the United States, though in other countries, such as England, patients can wait as long as a year for a procedure such as a hip replacement.[24]

The social responsibility for enabling the frail to flourish also extends to promoting the growth of suitable housing. Just as federal legislation stimulated the growth of nursing homes in the 1930s, Congress could spur construction of community housing designed to care for the frail elderly.[25] Simply building new facilities, however, will not be enough. Currently, new complexes are sprouting up throughout the country because running an assisted-living facility is profitable: only those who can afford to pay the thirty thousand dollars or more per year price tag are eligible.[26] To make assisted living a viable option for the majority of frail elderly, it will have to be financially feasible. Realistically, it will be affordable only if Medicaid or a new long-term care benefit within Medicare subsidizes part of the cost of assisted living.

Sustaining the frail so that they can lead satisfying lives will also require that Medicare develop a commitment to home care. Medicare reimbursement for home-care services has always been limited—restricted primarily to providing services during bouts of acute illness, especially after hospitalization. But expenditures on home care by Medicare began soaring in the 1990s as hospital stays became progressively shorter. The number of patients receiving Medicare home services doubled between 1989 and 1995, leading Congress to start tightening the screws on home-care services by passing the Balanced Budget Act.[27] Judging by the falling percentage of frail elders entering nursing homes, Medicare home services were effective: the home health aides who helped with personal care, homemakers who helped with household chores, and nurses and therapists who provided medical care and rehabilitation were making a difference in the lives of frail elders. If these individuals are to lead active lives, the kinds of lives that most wish to lead, they will need more assistance, not less.

A further role for government will be in regulating assisted-living facilities. Currently, such facilities are unregulated in many states and minimally regulated in most. As a consequence, there are no standards for how much on-site nursing care must be available, for how much training the aides who provide personal care must receive, or for what the nutritional content of the meals should be. Assisted-living facilities do not have to face frequent inspections by regulatory agencies looking for violations of a long list of rules. The absence of oversight is both liberating and dangerous. Like the "rest homes," or "board and care" homes, that preceded them, assisted-living facilities have the potential to offer the ideal combination of privacy and institutional support. The homey atmosphere of the old-fashioned rest homes was largely destroyed—or the homes put out of business altogether—by regulations requiring, for example, that a nurse be on the premises a specified number of hours each day and that special fire doors be installed. The concern was that without such rules, the personnel administering medication would be unaware of the potential side effects of the pills on the one hand, and the facilities would be fire traps on the other. In fact, there was evidence that the aides dispensing medications were unable to recognize medication toxicity when it occurred and that there were a number of instances of devastating fires in rest homes.[28] However, forcing mom-and-pop establishments to adhere to staffing and fire codes transformed many homes into institutions. Frail elders were protected from certain medical and physical mishaps, but their lives became more regimented, their environment more bureaucratic.[29] Assisted living faces the same dilemma: government will undoubtedly intervene with regulations to protect the vulnerable elderly. The challenge is to design regulations that achieve their goals without destroying the milieu of assisted living.

The responsible social response to frailty should also include creating medical institutions organized to provide the type of medical care that makes sense for the frail elderly. Many of the people described in this book, at some point in their course, opted for an approach to medical care midway between maximally aggressive and merely palliative. Some of their physicians were comfortable with this strategy, and others saw the options in more black-and-white terms.[30] Making intermediate treatment widely available to the frail elderly will necessitate more emphasis on geriatrics in medical schools and residency programs.[31] It will also require modifying the Medicare program—including altering senior HMOs that provide a growing fraction of the care to the elderly—to offer a set of benefits that reflect the distinctive priorities of many frail elders. A proposed program called MediCaring, for instance, would allow subscribers the option of more supportive services and more home services in exchange for fewer hospital benefits.[32] Such a system would encourage a person with pneumonia or an exacerbation of his chronic congestive heart failure to stay at home for treatment, forgoing more invasive treatment in return for greater comfort. Patients will make such a trade-off only if they can obtain the essentials of medical care at home, including adequate nursing care, intravenous medication, and oxygen.[33]

Access to assistive devices, better housing, and new insurance plans should constitute the core of the communal response to frailty. But for society to truly accept frailty as a stage of life—not an inevitable stage, but a phase for many, many people—and to embrace the frail as full-fledged members of that society, the dominant attitude toward the frail will have to be transformed.

Instead of viewing the frail as failures, individuals who have, through sloth or misfortune, lost their vigor and become dependent, the frail should simply be regarded as people with disabilities. The frail need both human and technical support to thrive as members of the community, just as others with disabilities need support. It is the responsibility of a just and compassionate society to guarantee that assistance, a step the society will be reluctant to take if the frail continue to be viewed chiefly as a burden.

For attitudes to change, we will need to abandon our relentless emphasis on productivity. Adults are typically valued for their contributions to their fields or the gross national product. Children are commonly valued as future adults: we accept the need to invest in them to ensure that they will become productive adults. The elderly are valued principally if they continue working, either at their old jobs or in new ones. Instead of seeking to re-create the old in the image of the middle-aged, we need to find a new image for them, especially for those who are frail. If the frail elderly are not likely to win respect from society by their economic contributions, they can garner respect through their roles as nurturers and counselors, instructors and assistants. Just as many women have rebelled against the strand of feminism that seeks to elevate the status of women solely by enabling them to pursue the same kinds of careers as men, so, too, should the elderly rebel against the tendency to equate a successful old age with continued productivity. Some feminists have argued that caregiving and other endeavors centered on relationships should be accorded equal status to traditional work. It is this type of activity, which is conventionally viewed as "women's work," that is eminently suitable to the frail elderly. Tutoring reading, as demonstrated by Peggy Simon, or extending herself to others, as exemplified by Catherine Endicott, are ways for the frail to find meaning in life. If society comes to esteem nurturing, if it creates opportunities for the elderly to play such roles, it will ultimately transform its image of the frail from passive, dependent, and superannuated to active, involved, and valued members of the community.

Over the next fifty years, the seventy-six million baby boomers born in the two decades following World War II will enter old age. By 2010 they will begin qualifying for Medicare, and twenty years later will swell the ranks of the frail. Current projections indicate that by 2040, there will be 14.4 million elderly Americans living at home who need help with their daily activities, including 2.8 million who have severe disabilities, and a doubling or tripling of the number of elderly people living in nursing homes.[34] These predictions may be an overstatement of just how dire the future will be. Families, policy-makers, and the elderly themselves should not be paralyzed by "apocalyptic demography."[35] We should neither assume that all old people are destined to be frail nor that they are certain to remain vigorous. Instead, we should craft a tripartite response to the *risk* of frailty—we need to develop strategies to help prevent frailty, to systematically prepare families and the medical system for dealing with frailty, and to enable the frail elderly to transcend their physical limitations.

Prevention includes encouraging the middle-aged of today to exercise, to seek treatment for depression, to vigorously treat high blood pressure, and to build strong friendship networks. It means educating physicians and employers to advocate interventions that have been shown to work, and beginning a lifelong education process for the general public, starting at the elementary school level. Promoting prevention also means supporting research investigating other approaches that have not yet been tested and that may contribute to avoiding or postponing frailty.

Preparation for frailty means creating the infrastructure necessary to allow older people to fulfill their potential. We will have to build on the patchwork of services and housing options already available to find ways to promote ongoing engagement with life, not merely to sustain existence. We should take advantage of technology to overcome some of the barriers preventing the frail elderly from flourishing. Creative solutions to the formidable problems involved in supporting rather than merely sustaining the frail elderly will require input from architects (to design suitable housing), computer scientists (to create interactive software to compensate for physical deficits), and art and music therapists (to identify and organize meaningful activities for frail elders to engage in), as well as from other professionals not traditionally identified with gerontology.

Once the necessary resources and institutions are in place, then those older people who, despite their efforts at prevention, become frail will find they can transcend their limitations. The frail elderly should be able to remain involved in the human community. Their involvement is likely to be different in kind and extent from their earlier involvement: it is more apt to be based on interpersonal interactions and less likely to center on productivity. It is likely to be a part-time rather than a full-time activity, given the extensive amount of time the elderly will continue to devote to basic self-care. But contrary to the once popular theory that older people disengage from life in their final years, even the frail elderly can continue to engage with life. The challenge—for individuals with frailty and their families and for society as a whole—is to enable the soul of every frail person to clap its hands and sing.

> *An aged man is but a paltry thing,*
> *A tattered coat upon a stick, unless*
> *Soul clap its hands and sing, and louder sing*
> *For every tatter in its mortal dress.* [36]

Sources and Resources

Information on aging in general and on frailty in particular can be obtained through the following sources:

American Society on Aging
833 Market Street, Suite 501
San Francisco, CA 94103
415-974-9600
This nonprofit organization of professionals working in the field of aging sponsors conferences and publishes the magazine *Aging Today*.
http://www.asaging.org/

American Association of Retired Persons (AARP)
601 East Street, NW
Washington, DC 20049
1-800-424-3410

This private nonprofit organization publishes information on a
variety of issues related to aging, including insurance, exercise, and
diet. It publishes the magazine *Modern Maturity.*
http://www.aarp.org

American Association of Homes and Services for the Aging
901 East Street, NW, Suite 500
Washington, DC 20004-2011
202-783-2242
This organization seeks to promote a comprehensive system of care
and services that recognizes the dignity of all persons and enhances
the quality of life for older adults.
http://www.aahsa.org/

Gerontological Society of America
1030 15th Street, NW, Suite 250
Washington, DC 20005-1503
202-842-1275
This multidisciplinary national organization of professionals in the
field of aging publishes a magazine and sponsors an annual conference about aging. Its mission is to promote the scientific study of
aging and to foster the use of gerontologic research in forming
public policy.
http://www.geron.org/

Novartis Foundation for Gerontology
S-200. 2.97, Lichtstrasse
CH-4002 Basel, Switzerland
Telephone number: 41 61 3247421
This foundation maintains an educational Web site to provide
interaction between health-care professionals and the public. It
offers information on topics such as depression, impaired mobility,
and incontinence.
http://www.healthandage.com/

National Institute on Aging
Information Center
PO Box 8057
Gaithersburg, MD 20892-2296
1-800-222-2225
The NIA is the principal biomedical research agency that promotes healthy aging by conducting and supporting research. It also offers written material for the general public on various medical conditions afflicting the elderly.
http://www.nih.gov/nia

Administration on Aging of the U.S. Department of Health and Human Services
330 Independence Avenue, SW
Washington, DC 20201
This agency works with state and local agencies on aging to develop and coordinate community services for the elderly. It provides a resource directory for older people and fact sheets on a variety of topics for professionals in the field of aging, service providers, and older Americans and their families.
http://www.aoa.dhhs.gov/

NOTES

Introduction: Frailty in Our Time

1. J. Fries, "Aging, Natural Death, and the Compression of Morbidity," *New England Journal of Medicine* 303 (1980): 130–5. Dr. Fries was the main proponent of the view that advances in health care have led to a "compression of morbidity."

2. L. Verbrugge, "Longer Life but Worsening Health? Trends in Health and Mortality of Middle-aged and Older Persons," *Milbank Memorial Fund Quarterly* 62 (1984): 475–519.

3. There is no universally agreed-upon definition of frailty. The formulation here is similar to what is found in I. Brown, R. Resnick, and D. Raphael, "Frailty: Constructing a Common Meaning, Definition, and Conceptual Framework," in the *Journal of Rehabilitation Research* 18 (1995): 93–102. For an attempt to understand the biological basis of frailty, see D. Hamerman, "Toward an Understanding of Frailty," *Annals of Internal Medicine* 130 (1999): 945–50.

4. See K. Manton, L. Corder, and E. Stallard, "Chronic Disability Trends in Elderly United States Population, 1982–1994," *Proceedings of the National Academy of Sciences* 94 (1997): 2553–8. This study reported that the prevalence of disability in the elderly was down 3.6 percent.

5. J. Guralnik and E. Simonsick, "Physical Disability in Older Americans," *Gerontology* 48 (1993): 3–10.

6. One way of looking at the question of the duration of frailty has been to measure its inverse, or "active life expectancy." This is the number of years remaining during which an individual is independent. At age eighty-five, men have a life expectancy of 5.11 years, an active life expectancy of 2.55 years, and an expected 0.84 years in an institution. The corresponding numbers for women at age eighty-five are a life expectancy of 6.44 years, an active life expectancy of 2.25 years, and an anticipated 1.69 years in an institution. See K. Manton, E. Stallard, and L. Corder, "Changes in Morbidity and Chronic Disability in the U.S. Elderly Population. Evidence from the 1982, 1984, and 1989 National Long Term Care Surveys," *Journal of Gerontology* 50 (1995): S194–204.

7. U.S. Senate Special Committee on Aging. *Aging America: Trends and Projections.* U.S. Department of Health and Human Services. Washington, D.C., 1988.

Chapter 1: The Roads to Frailty

1. For a brilliant essay on the transformation induced in large measure by the germ theory of disease, see Charles Rosenberg, "The Therapeutic Revolution: Medicine, Meaning, and Social Change in Nineteenth-Century America," in Charles Rosenberg, *Explaining Epidemics and Other Studies in the History of Medicine* (New York: Cambridge University Press, 1992), 9–31.

2. The course is not invariably downhill. Approximately one-fourth of elderly individuals living at home who are dependent at any given point in time will have recovered their independence in the next fifteen months. L. Branch, S. Katz, K. Kriegman, and J. Papsidero, "A Prospective Study of Functional Status Among Community Elders," *American Journal of Public Health* 74 (1984): 266–8.

3. The paths to frailty, or the disablement process, has been formally studied. In those over eighty-five, progressive disability accounts for more than half of the cases of frailty, as opposed to catastrophic disability. The mortality rate is high in both types, with a median survival of 3.4 years in women and 2.1 years in men. L. Ferrucci, J. Guralnik, E. Simonsick et al., "Progressive Versus Catastrophic Disability: A Longitudinal View of the Disablement Process," *Journal of Gerontology* 51 (1996): M123–30.

4. J. Croft, W. Giles, R. Pollard et al., "Heart Failure Survival Among Older Adults in the United States: A Poor Prognosis for an Emerging Epidemic in the Medicare Population," *Archives of Internal Medicine* 159 (1999): 505–10. This study looked at the survival rate of older adults after their first hospitalization for heart failure in 1986. Only 19 percent of black men, 16 percent of white men, 25 percent of black women, and 23 percent of white women survived six years. Medical treatment of congestive heart failure has improved since 1986, but another study that looked at nursing home patients over the age of eighty who were hospitalized for CHF between 1989 and 1995 found that 61 percent were dead within a year. See R. Wang, M. Mouliswar, S. Denman, and M. Kleban, "Mortality of Institutionalized Old-Old Hospitalized with Congestive Heart Failure," *Archives of Internal Medicine* 158 (1998): 2464–8.

5. M. Tinetti, M. Speechley, and S. Ginter, "Risk Factors for Falls Among Elderly Persons Living in the Community," *New England Journal of Medicine* 322 (1990): 286–90.

6. Tremendous progress has been made in the treatment of heart attacks, but heart disease is still the number one cause of death in adults. See D. Davis, G. Dinse, and D. Hoel, "Decreasing Cardiovascular Disease and Increasing Cancer Among Whites in the United States from 1973 through 1987," *Journal of the American Medical Association* 271 (1994): 431–7. Between 1973 and 1987, cardiovascular mortality fell 42 percent in those aged fifty-five to eighty-four.

7. Stroke is the third leading cause of death in adults. (U.S. Senate Special Committee on Aging. *Aging in America: Trends and Projections.* U.S. Department of Health and Human Services. Washington D.C., 1988.) Even more important for the discussion here, stroke is a leading cause of functional limitation in the elderly. C. Boult, R. Kane, T. Louis et al., "Chronic Conditions that Lead to Functional Limitation in the Elderly," *Gerontology* 49 (1994): M28–36, found that arthritis and cerebrovascular disease were the best predictors of the development of limitation of function. Stroke comes in several varieties: thrombotic stroke (in which a blood vessel to the brain is blocked, usually from atherosclerosis), embolic stroke (in which a blood vessel in the brain is blocked because a clot traveled from elsewhere in the body, typically the heart), and hemorrhagic stroke (in which a blood vessel bursts and blood leaks into the brain tissue).

8. Parkinson's disease is a progressive neurologic disorder with three main symptoms: stiffness, tremor, and slowness of movement. In about a third of cases it is associated with depression, and, similarly, in about a third of cases (not necessarily the same third) dementia develops. The vast majority of cases of Parkinson's disease are "idiopathic," i.e., the cause is unknown, though we do know what goes wrong: the part of the brain responsible for the production of the neurotransmitter dopamine is damaged and inadequate amounts of dopamine are made. Parkinson's disease can now be treated, principally by dopamine replacement, but the progressive nature of the disease means that treatment becomes less effective over time.

9. Depression will be discussed later in this book. A well-written book about suicide in general is K. Jamison's *Night Falls Fast: Understanding Suicide* (New York: Knopf, 1999).

Chapter 2: Fixing the Fixable Part

1. Disengagement theory was put forth by Elaine Cumming and William Henry in their book, *Growing Old* (New York: Basic Books, 1961). It has since then been largely discredited. See J. Bell, "Disengagement Versus Engagement—A Need for Greater Expectations," *Journal of the American Geriatric Society* 26 (1978): 89–95; and also W. Achenbaum and V. Bengtson, "Re-engaging the Disengagement Theory of Aging: On the History and Assessment Theory Development in Gerontology," *Gerontologist* 34 (1994): 756–63.

2. Benign prostatic hyperplasia is almost universal in elderly men. In the presence of severe symptoms—such as the inability to void—surgery is routinely recommended. In fact, four hundred thousand transurethral prostatectomies are performed in the United States each year, making it the second most common operation in the elderly after cataract extraction. For more moderate symptoms, medication is available, including finasteride and terazosin. Other therapies, such as microwave treatments, can also be helpful. See J. Oesterling, "Benign Prostatic Hyperplasia. Medical and Minimally Invasive Treatment Options," *New England Journal of Medicine* 332 (1995): 99–109.

3. Cancer is the second leading cause of death in older people. Lung cancer is the leading cause of death from malignancy among men. (U.S. Senate Special Committee on Aging. *Aging America: Trends and Projections*. U.S. Department of Health and Human Services. Washington, D.C., 1988.)

4. J. Nadol, "Hearing Loss," *New England Journal of Medicine* 379 (1993): 1092–102.

5. R. Lavizzo-Mourey and E. Siegler, "Hearing Impairment in the Elderly," *Journal of General Internal Medicine* 7 (1992): 191–8.

6. C. Mulrow, "Quality-of-Life Changes and Hearing Impairment. A Randomized Trial," *Annals of Internal Medicine* 113 (1990): 188–94.

7. See U.S. Senate Special Committee on Aging, op. cit. Ischemic heart disease is also one of seven conditions that have a major impact on function. The others are arthritis, visual impairment, decreased hearing, chronic lung disease, diabetes, and cancer. See L. Verbrugge and D. Patrick, "Seven Chronic Conditions: Their Impact on U.S. Adults' Activity Levels and Use of Medical Services," *American Journal of Public Health* 85 (1995): 173–82.

8. Between 1980 and 1990, the death rate from heart disease fell 34 percent. Approximately 25 percent of the decline can be attributed to primary prevention (decreasing the rate of heart disease in the first place by decreased rates of cigarette smoking, for example), and another 29 percent is attributed to reduction in risk factors in patients with known coronary disease. The rest of the decline is presumably due to improvements in treatment. See M. Hunink, L. Goldman, A. Tosteson et al., "The Recent Decline in Mortality from Coronary Heart Disease, 1980–1990," *Journal of the American Medical Association* 277 (1997): 535–42.

9. Angioplasty is successful 90 percent of the time in opening up a coronary artery that is not totally blocked. It provides relief of angina in most patients with just one affected coronary artery. See C. Landau, R. Lange, and L. Hillis, "Percutaneous Transluminal Coronary Angioplasty," *New England Journal of Medicine* 330 (1994): 981–93.

10. D. Fischman, M. Leon, D. Baim et al., "A Randomized Comparison of Coronary-Stent Placement and Balloon Angioplasty in the Treatment of Coronary Artery Disease," *New England Journal of Medicine* 331 (1994): 496–501. This study found that stents per-

formed slightly better than angioplasty: there was a higher rate of short-term success, and after six months, the stented lesions had a larger diameter and a lower rate of re-stenosis. The re-stonosis rates were quite high in both groups: 32 percent with stents, compared to 42 percent with angioplasty.

11. The thirty-day mortality in the elderly fell 37 percent after angioplasty and 18 percent after CABG during the period 1987–90. During the same period, one-year mortality fell 22 percent and 19 percent, respectively. See E. Peterson, J. Jollis, J. Bebchuk et al., "Changes in Mortality after Myocardial Revascularization in the Elderly," *Annals of Internal Medicine* 121 (1994): 919–27.

12. J. Ernest, "Changes and Diseases of the Aging Eye," in C. Cassel, H. Cohen, E. Larson et al., *Geriatrics*, 3rd ed. (New York: Springer, 1997), 683–97.

13. See "Vision Problems in the United States," Schaumburg, Il.: *Preventing Blindness America*, 1994.

14. The risk of developing a gastrointestinal complication such as a bleeding ulcer is increased approximately fivefold in elderly people taking nonsteroidal anti-inflammatory medication. See S. Gabriel, L. Jaakkimainen, and C. Bomardier, "Risk for Serious Gastrointestinal Complications Related to Use of Nonsteroidal Anti-inflammatory Drugs," *Annals of Internal Medicine* 115 (1991): 787–92.

15. Not only is arthritis number one, it is extraordinarily widespread. In people over age eighty-five living at home, 66 percent of men and 74 percent of women report they have arthritis. See K. Manton, E. Stallard, and L. Corder, "Changes in Morbidity and Chronic Disability in the U.S. Elderly Population: Evidence from the 1982, 1984, and 1989 National Long Term Care Surveys," *Gerontology* 50B (1995): S194–S204.

16. A new kind of nonsteroidal anti-inflammatory medication is now available—the COX-2 inhibitors. These include rofecoxib (brand

name Vioxx) and celecoxib (brand name Celebrex). These drugs were approved by the Federal Drug Administration for treatment of osteoarthritis. Recent studies indicate that these agents are as effective as older nonsteroidal anti-inflammatory drugs, but with fewer side effects. See M. Langman, D. Jensen, D. Watson, et al., "Adverse Upper Gastro-intestinal Effects of Rofecoxib Compared with NSAIDS," *Journal of the American Medical Association* 282 (1999): 1929–1933.

17. NIH Consensus Development Panel on Total Hip Replacement, "Total Hip Replacement," *Journal of the American Medical Association* 273 (1995): 1950–6.

Chapter 3: The Moves Make the Man

1. An early discussion of the meaning of prospective payment for hospitals under Medicare, also known as diagnosis-related groups, is found in B. Vladeck, "Medicare Hospital Payment of Diagnosis-Related Groups," *Annals of Internal Medicine* (1984): 576–581. A more recent discussion of the Medicare program in general, also authored by Bruce Vladeck, the former director of the Health Care Financing Administration, the agency that runs Medicare, is B. Vladeck and K. King, "Medicare at 30: Preparing for the Future," *Journal of the American Medical Association* 274 (1995): 259–62.

2. The Balanced Budget Act will produce the most dramatic changes in the Medicare program since its inception in 1965. Over the next five years, it mandates a $16.2 billion cut in funding for home health care. See W. Ettinger, "The Balanced Budget Act of 1997: Implications for the Practice of Geriatric Medicine," *Journal of the American Geriatrics Society* 46 (1998): 530–3.

3. A good summary of what is covered by Medicare and Medicaid can be found in N. DeLew, "The First 30 Years of Medicare and Med-

icaid," *Journal of the American Medical Association* 274 (1995): 262–7. Since the details change frequently, the most up-to-date information can be obtained from the Web page of the Health Care Financing Administration, the agency that runs the Medicare program: http://www.hcfa.gov.

4. For more information on how regulations affect quality of life in nursing homes, see M. Gillick, "The Role of the Rules: The Impact of the Bureaucratization of Long-Term Care," in S. Toombs, D. Barnard, and R. Carson, eds., *Chronic Illness: From Experience to Policy* (Bloomington, Ind.: Indiana University Press, 1995), 189–211.

5. Osteoporosis is defined as a disorder in which there is low bone mass. It most commonly affects the wrist, spine, hip, and upper arm. Many treatments are now available, including estrogen and medication known as bisphosphonates. See R. Eastell, "Treatment of Postmenopausal Osteoporosis," *New England Journal of Medicine* 338 (1998): 736–46.

6. For a discussion of the ways that nursing homes can be made better places for older people to live in, see M. Gillick, "Long-Term Care Options for the Frail Elderly," *Journal of the American Geriatrics Society* 37 (1989): 1198–203.

Chapter 4: When Acute Illness Strikes

1. A study by M. Danis, D. Patrick, L. Southerland, and M. Green, "Patients' and Families' Preferences for Medical Intensive Care," *Journal of the American Medical Association* 260 (1988): 797–802, interviewed elderly survivors of an ICU stay, or their families in the cases where the patients did not survive. The authors found that 70 percent of patients and families were willing to undergo intensive care again to achieve as little as one month's survival. Only 8 per-

cent were unwilling to undergo intensive care regardless of how long their survival could be increased. It is important to recognize that the only patients interviewed in this study had survived the experience. For those who died, family members were interviewed who might well have been reluctant to say they wished their relatives had never been in the ICU.

2. T. Fried and M. Gillick, "Medical Decision-Making in the Last Six Months of Life: Choices about Limitations of Care," *Journal of the American Geriatrics Society* 42 (1994): 303–7.

3. See T. Fried, M. Gillick, and L. Lipsitz, "Short-Term Functional Outcomes of Long-Term Care Residents with Pneumonia Treated with and without Hospital Transfer," *Journal of the American Geriatrics Society* 45 (1997): 302–6. In the specific case of pneumonia, for example, patients transferred from a nursing home to an acute hospital for treatment were more likely to experience further loss of independence than were otherwise similar patients who were treated in the nursing home. Another study, which looked at very ill hospitalized patients with any of nine different medical conditions, found that two months after hospitalization, the number of people with limitations in their daily activities tripled. The strongest predictor of who would develop severe limitations was who had limitations prior to the hospitalization. See A. Wu, A. Damiano, J. Lynn et al., "Predicting Future Functional Status for Seriously Ill Hospitalized Adults: The SUPPORT Prognostic Model," *Annals of Internal Medicine* 122 (1995): 342–50.

4. One of the earliest—and clearest—descriptions of delirium is by Z. Lipowski, "Delirium (Acute Confusional States)," *Journal of the American Medical Association* 258 (1987): 1789–92. Lipowski reported that delirium affected 30 to 50 percent of hospitalized patients over the age of seventy.

5. Most studies do not consider frailty as a factor to be considered in assessing the efficacy of treatment; they tend to look at how sick

people are and at co-morbidities (other medical conditions). A recent study that did consider physical and cognitive function at baseline found that older people with the poorest ratings on scores of physical and mental function had a 60 percent in-hospital mortality, compared to a 20 percent mortality for those with the highest physical- and mental-function scores. See S. Inouye, P. Peduzzi, S. Robison et al., "Importance of Functional Measures in Predicting Mortality Among Older Hospitalized Patients," *Journal of the American Medical Association* 279 (1998): 1187–93.

6. For a review of a number of studies on the effectiveness of gastrostomy tubes in preventing aspiration pneumonia, see T. Finucane and J. Bynum, "Use of Tube Feeding to Prevent Aspiration Pneumonia," *Lancet* 348 (1996): 1421–4.

7. In a fairly large study of survival among patients over age seventy undergoing CPR, D. Murphy, A. Murray, B. Robinson, and E. Campion found that only 3.8 percent of people with a cardiac arrest survived to be discharged from a hospital. The survival rate for those who had an arrest outside an acute-care hospital and were transferred to the hospital was only 0.8 percent: "Outcome of Cardiopulmonary Resuscitation in the Elderly," *Annals of Internal Medicine* 111 (1989): 199–205.

8. This is the second time BPH has made an appearance in these pages. Ben Frank also had BPH and, in fact, developed urinary retention—the inability to go to the bathroom on his own—after he started taking an antidepressant.

9. C. Fleming, J. Wasson, P. Albertsen et al., for the Prostate Outcomes Research Team, "A Decision Analysis of Alternative Treatment Strategies for Clinically Localized Prostate Cancer," *Journal of the American Medical Association* 269 (1993): 2650–8. This analysis suggested that radical prostatectomy and radiotherapy would benefit people with localized cancer, especially younger patients with "high-grade" tumors (determined by examining the cells under a

microscope). Watchful waiting was a reasonable alternative for men with localized prostate cancer. Subsequent studies have confirmed this finding, arguing that 87 percent of men will have a ten-year disease-free survival if their tumors are low-grade and no therapy is performed. See G. Chodak, R. Thisted, G. Gerber et al., "Results of Conservative Management of Clinically Localized Prostate Cancer, *New England Journal of Medicine* 330 (1994): 242–8.

10. Many authorities advise against screening when they use quality-adjusted life expectancy to measure outcomes. See M. Krahn, J. Mahoney, M. Eichman et al., "Screening for Prostate Cancer. A Decision Analytic View," *Journal of the American Medical Association* 272 (1994): 773–80.

11. W. Catalone, "Management of Cancer of the Prostate," *New England Journal of Medicine* 331 (1996): 996–1003, recommends hormonal therapy as an option for men with localized disease, especially older men.

12. The study was done by D. Berggren, Y. Gustafson, Y. Eriksson et al., "Acute Confusional States in Elderly Patients Treated for Femoral Neck Fracture," *Journal of the American Geriatrics Society* 36 (1988): 525–30.

13. Pneumonia/influenza is the fifth leading cause of death in the elderly (based on death-certificate data). See F. Schick and R. Schick, eds., *Statistical Handbook on Aging Americans* (Phoenix, Ariz.: Oryx Press, 1994), 135.

14. *Radical* is the technical term for the operation, not a pejorative description. It is radical because it involves removal of surrounding lymph nodes and other tissues. It is, not surprisingly, radical in its physiological consequences as well: it frequently produces impotence and incontinence.

15. Roman Catholicism, a religious tradition that believes strongly in the sanctity of life, and that tends to favor life-sustaining treatment,

makes clear that such treatment is required only if "the benefits outweigh the burdens involved to the patient." (National Conference of Catholic Bishops, "Ethical and Religious Directives for Catholic Health Care Services," Washington, D.C., 1995.) Orthodox Judaism, which likewise places a heavy emphasis on preserving life, rejects interventions that cause or prolong suffering. Many authorities argue against "impediments to dying." See R. Schostak, "Jewish Ethical Guidelines for Resuscitation and Artificial Nutrition of the Dying Elderly," *Journal of Medical Ethics* 20 (1994): 93–100.

Chapter 5: Not by Bread Alone

1. See C. Arensberg and A. Niehoff, "American Cultural Values," in J. Spradley and M. Rynkiewich, eds., *The Nacirema* (Boston: Little, Brown, 1975). The survey on which this conclusion is based was done in the early 1970s, but the view that people are judged by their work, their ability to earn a living, is echoed ten years later in the work of R. Bellah, R. Madsen, W. Sullivan et al., *Habits of the Heart: Individualism and Commitment in American Life* (New York: Harper & Row, 1986). This study found that middle-class Americans believed that meaning stemmed from the acquisition of wealth, status, and authority, although many people, in fact, found meaning in "communities of memory," such as religious or cultural groups.

2. Betty Friedan, *The Fountain of Age* (New York: Simon & Schuster, 1993).

3. The numbers are so large as to be almost meaningless. Perhaps more useful is the observation that a total of $108 billion was spent on long-term care for the elderly in the United States in 1993: $44 billion paid for by Medicaid, $15 billion by Medicare, $9 billion

by miscellaneous sources, and $39 billion out of pocket by the elderly themselves (*36 percent of the total*). See B.Vladeck, N. Miller, and S. Clauser, "The Changing Face of Long-Term Care," *Health Care Financing Review* 14 (1993): 5–23.

4. A good book about saying good-bye is Ira Byock, *Dying Well* (New York: Riverhead Press, 1997).

5. The special kind of autonomy involved in implementing a decision, rather than merely in making the decision, has been called *executional autonomy*, as distinguished from *decisional autonomy*. The frail person knows what he wants and can make plans, but requires others to carry out his plans. See G. Agich, "Actual Autonomy and Long-Term Care Decision-Making," in L. McCullough and N. Wilson, eds., *Long-Term Care Decisions. Ethical and Conceptual Issues* (Baltimore: Johns Hopkins University Press, 1995), 113–36. See also B. Collopy, "Autonomy and Long-Term Care: Some Cultural Distinctions," *Gerontologist* 28 (1988): 10–17.

6. For the two different historical perspectives, see W. A. Achenbaum, *Old Age in the New Land* (Baltimore: Johns Hopkins University Press, 1978), and David Fischer, *Growing Old in America* (New York: Oxford University Press, 1978).

7. Changes in attitudes toward old age are described in Thomas Cole's book survey of the history of the view of old age in the West, *The Journey of Life* (Cambridge, Mass.: Cambridge University Press, 1991).

8. A discussion of the joys and the miseries of caregiving for individuals with dementia is found in A. Motenko, "The Frustrations, Satisfactions, and Well-being of Dementia Caregivers," *Gerontologist* 29 (1989): 166–72. A three-part series on caregiving appeared in New York *Newsday* in April 1995, written by Laura Muha. She cites the statistics that 14 percent of men and 26 percent of women over eighty-five live with adult children and that more than *25 million* people care for elderly relatives in the United States today.

9. There is a large and growing literature on caregiving. Elaine Brody's book, *Women in the Middle: The Parent-Care Years* (New York: Springer, 1990), discusses the difficulties encountered by working women.

10. A fascinating account of the basis of memory is D. Schachter, *Searching for Memory: The Brain, the Mind, and the Past* (New York: Basic Books, 1996).

11. For more on these rituals, plus those of Muslims and Buddhists, see J. Neuberger, "Cultural Issues in Palliative Care," in D. Doyle, G. Hanks, and N. MacDonald, eds., *Oxford Textbook of Palliative Medicine* (New York: Oxford University Press, 1998), 777–85.

12. A major proponent of this view is Ronald Dworkin. See, for example, his article "Autonomy and the Demented Self," *Milbank Quarterly* 64 (suppl. 2) 1986: 4–16.

13. It is no accident that three out of the four characters in this book spent at least some time in a nursing home. Current projections are that of the 2.2 million people who turned sixty-five in 1990, 43 percent are expected to enter a nursing home at least once before death. The risk is much higher in those who become frail. The length of stay in the nursing home is variable, as is the case in this book: one-third can expect to spend at least three months, 24 percent at least one year, and 9 percent at least five years. See P. Kemper and C. Murtaugh, "Lifetime Use of Nursing Home Care," *New England Journal of Medicine* 324 (1991): 595–603.

14. J. Avorn and E. Langer, "Induced Disability in Nursing Home Patients: A Controlled Trial," *Journal of the American Geriatrics Society* 30 (1982): 397–400.

15. R. Kane, A. Caplan, E. Urv-Wong et al., "Everyday Matters in the Lives of Nursing Home Residents: Wish for and Perception of Choice and Control," *Journal of the American Geriatrics Society* 45 (1997): 1086–93. In this study, 135 nursing home residents living

in 25 different nursing homes were asked what was important to them. Most important were bedtime, rising time, food, roommates, use of the telephone, trips out of the nursing home, and initiating contact with a physician.

16. H. Feldman, I. Goldstein, D. Hatzichristou et al., "Impotence and its Medical and Psychosocial Correlates: Results of the Massachusetts Male Aging Study," *Journal of Urology* 151 (1994): 54–61. Data on men over eighty is harder to come by, but the Baltimore Longitudinal Study of Aging, a study of healthy, community-dwelling elders, reported impotence occurring in 75 percent of eighty-year-olds.

17. A. Halgason, J. Adolfsson, P. Dickman et al., "Factors Associated with Waning Sexual Function among Elderly Men and Prostate Cancer Patients," *Journal of Urology* 158 (1997): 155–9.

18. M. Ehrenfeld, G. Bronner, N. Tabak et al., "Sexuality Among Institutionalized Elderly Patients with Dementia," *Nursing Ethics* 6 (1999): 144–9. In general, nursing home staff and family members of residents accept amorous but not erotic involvement among nursing home residents.

19. An inspiring testimonial to the capacity of the human spirit to triumph over extreme disability and galloping frailty is Mitch Albom's *Tuesdays with Morrie* (New York: Doubleday, 1997). Albom relates a series of interviews with his former sociology professor, Morrie Schwartz, who at seventy-eight is diagnosed with amyotrophic lateral sclerosis. Schwartz rapidly loses the use of his hands. In what he regards as a major blow to his dignity, he stops being able to wipe himself. Ultimately, he develops difficulty breathing and can speak only in short bursts. He dies of respiratory failure as the nerves to successive muscles fail. His student discusses with him what gives meaning to life: family, passionate engagement with the world, intimacy, and giving to the community.

20. This is consistent with what Sharon Kaufman found, as reported in her book *The Ageless Self: Sources of Meaning in Later Life* (Madison, Wisc.: University of Wisconsin Press, 1986).

21. Ernest Becker, *The Denial of Death* (New York: The Free Press, 1973).

22. Erik Erikson, *Childhood and Society* (New York: W. W. Norton & Co., 1963), describes the eight stages of the life cycle.

23. Sharon Kaufman, op. cit., 161.

Chapter 6: Facing Frailty: Prevention and Social Responsibility

1. J. Guralnick and E. Simonsick, "Physical Disability in Older Americans," *Gerontology* 48 (1993): 3–10.

2. These statistics are from H. Koenig, D. Blazer, and L. Hocking, "Depression, Anxiety, and Other Affective Disorders," in the geriatrics textbook by C. Cassel, H. Cohen, E. Larson et al., eds., *Geriatric Medicine,* 3rd ed. (New York: Springer, 1997), 135.

3. See C. Reynolds, E. Frank, J. Perel et al., "Nortriptyline and Interpersonal Psychotherapy As Maintenance Therapies for Recurrent Major Depression: A Randomized Controlled Trial in Patients Older than 59 Years," *Journal of the American Medical Association* 281 (1999): 39–45.

4. See S. Wannamethee, A. Shaper, and M. Walker, "Changes in Physical Activity, Mortality, and Incidence of Coronary Heart Disease in Older Men," *Lancet* 351 (1998): 1603–8. Light or moderate physical activity lowered mortality. Similar findings regarding women were reported by L. Kushi, R. Fee, A. Folsom et al., "Physical Activity and Mortality in Post-Menopausal Women," *Journal of the American Medical Association* 277 (1997): 1287–92.

5. S. Wolf, H. Barnhart, N. Kutner et al., "Reducing Fractures and Falls in Older Persons: An Investigation of Tai Chi and Computerized Balance Training," *Journal of the American Geriatrics Society* 44 (1996): 489–97.

6. G. Erikssen, K. Listol, J. Bjornholt et al., "Changes in Physical Fitness and Changes in Mortality," *Lancet* 352 (1998): 759–62.

7. M. Fiatarone, E. O'Neill, H. Ryan et al., "Exercise Training and Nutritional Supplementation for Physical Frailty in Very Elderly People," *New England Journal of Medicine* 330 (1994): 1769–71.

8. Some authorities claim that the second most common form of dementia is "Lewy Body disease," a disorder that has some features of Parkinson's disease and some of Alzheimer's disease. This remains controversial, with many experts continuing to regard vascular dementia as the cause of about 20 percent of cases of dementia.

9. J. Forette, M. Seux, J. Stresser et al., "Prevention of Dementia in Randomised Double Blind Placebo-Controlled Systolic Hypertension in Europe (Syst-Eur) Trial," *Lancet* 352 (1998): 1342–51.

10. D. Snowdon, L. Greiner, J. Mortimer et al., "Brain Infarction and the Clinical Expression of Alzheimer Disease: The Nun Study," *Journal of the American Medical Association* 277 (1997): 813–17. Participants in the study were members of the School Sisters of Notre Dame. They lived in convents in the midwestern, eastern, and southern United States. All agreed to psychological testing during life and to donate their brains at the time of death. They were remarkable for sharing a standardized environment. Among the sixty-one participants who met criteria for Alzheimer's disease at autopsy, those who also had evidence of strokes had poorer cognitive function than those without strokes.

11. L. Berkman, L. Leo-Summers, and R. Horwitz, "Emotional Support and Survival after Myocardial Infarction. A Prospective, Popu-

lation-Based Study of the Elderly," *Annals of Internal Medicine* 117 (1992): 1003–9.

12. P. Kimmel, R. Peterson, K. Weeks et al., "Psychosocial Factors, Behavioral Compliance, and Survival in Urban Hemodialysis Patients," *Kidney International* 54 (1998): 245–54.

13. See V. Wilcox, S. Kasl, and L. Berkman, "Social Support and Physical Disability in Older People after Hospitalization: A Prospective Study," *Health Psychology* 13 (1994): 170–9. This study looked at patients with hip fractures, strokes, or heart attacks.

14. See G. Roth, D. Ingram, and M. Lane, "Caloric Restriction in Primates: Will It Work and How Will We Know?" *Journal of the American Geriatrics Society* 47 (1999): 896–903.

15. L. Hayflick, *How and Why We Age* (New York: Ballantine, 1994).

16. M. Sano, C. Ernesto, R. Thomas et al., "A Controlled Trial of Selegeline, Alpha-tocopherol, or Both As Treatment for Alzheimer's Disease. The Alzheimer's Disease Cooperative Study," *New England Journal of Medicine* 336 (1997): 1216–22. Alpha-tocopherol is vitamin E.

17. M. Diaz, B. Frei, J. Vita, and J. Keaney, "Antioxidants and Atherosclerotic Heart Disease," *New England Journal of Medicine* 337 (1997): 408–16.

18. L. Speroff, J. Rowan, J. Symons et al., "The Comparative Effect on Bone Density, Endometrium, and Lipids of Continuous Hormones As Replacement Therapy (CHART Study). A Randomized Controlled Trial," *Journal of the American Medical Association* 276 (1996): 1397–1403.

19. One study found that the risk of coronary heart disease in women taking estrogen was just about cut in half. See M. Stampfer, G. Colditz, W. Willett et al., "Postmenopausal Estrogen Therapy and Cardiovascular Disease. Ten-Year Follow-Up from the Nurses'

Health Study," *New England Journal of Medicine* 325 (1991): 756–62.

20. S. Shaywitz, B. Shaywitz, K. Pugh et al., "Effect of Estrogen on Brain Activity Patterns in Postmenopausal Women During Working Memory Tasks," *Journal of the American Medical Association* 281 (1999): 1197–202.

21. E. Barrett-Connor and D. Keritz-Silverstein, "Estrogen Replacement Therapy and Cognitive Function in Older Women," *Journal of the American Medical Association* 269 (1993): 2637–41.

22. These "designer estrogens," such as the drug raloxifene, have an antiestrogen effect on the reproductive organs. That is, they work like tamoxifen, a drug that blocks the effect of estrogen and is useful in treating breast cancer. The effect of drugs such as raloxifene on the brain is not yet established. See W. Khovidhunkit and D. Shobach, "Clinical Effects of Raloxifene Hydrochloride in Women," *Annals of Internal Medicine* 130 (1999): 431–9.

23. For more information on possible strategies for preventing frailty, see J. Rowe and R. Kahn, *Successful Aging* (New York: Pantheon Books, 1998), and also T. Perls, M. Silver, with J. Lauerman, *Living to 100: Lessons in Living to Your Maximum Potential at Any Age* (New York: Basic Books, 1999). A helpful compendium of information about aging is C. Cassel, ed., *The Practical Guide to Aging: What Everyone Needs to Know* (New York: New York University Press, 1999).

24. In England, under the National Health Service, the waiting time for elective procedures has been gradually falling. A study done in 1990 showed that the proportion of patients waiting more than a year for a total hip replacement fell from 14 percent to 4 percent between 1981 and 1986. See R. Rajartnam, N. Black, and M. Dalziel, "Total Hip Replacement in the National Health Services: Is the Need Being Met?" *Journal of Public Health Medicine* 12 (1990): 56–9.

25. The Social Security Act of 1935 prohibited the payment of social security to residents of public institutions, such as almshouses. This spurred the creation of private nursing homes to provide custodial care for the elderly. The Hill-Burton Act of 1954 provided congressional funds for construction of hospitals, including nursing homes modeled along the lines of hospitals. Between 1940 and 1970, the percentage of institutionalized elders living in nursing homes rose from 34 to 72. See M. Holstein and T. Cole, "Long-Term Care: A Historical Reflection," in L. McCullough and N. Wilson, eds., *Long-Term Care Decisions. Ethical and Conceptual Dimensions* (Baltimore: Johns Hopkins University Press, 1995), 15–34.

26. A very small number of facilities accept a very small number of people who are on Medicaid, the insurance program for the poor. Medicare and, increasingly, Medicaid see themselves as health-care programs, although nursing home care, which is paid for by Medicaid only for those who meet the means test, is primarily custodial.

27. H. Welch, D. Wennberg, and W. Welch, "The Use of Medicare Home Care Services," *New England Journal of Medicine* 335 (1996): 324–9.

28. J. Avorn, P. Dreyer, K. Connelly, and S. Soumerai, "Use of Psychoactive Medications and the Quality of Care in Rest Homes," *New England Journal of Medicine* 320 (1989): 227–32. Roughly half the staff at rest homes did not know that the medication haloperidol, widely used in the residents at the rest homes, could cause parkinsonian symptoms.

29. See E. Goffman, *Asylums: Essays on the Social Situation of Mental Patients and Other Inmates* (New York: Doubleday, 1961), for a discussion of "total institutions." Goffman characterizes institutions established to care for persons felt to be incapable and harmless (including homes for the aged) as analogous to mental hospitals, jails, and prisoner-of-war camps. He points out that in such facilities, each phase of the resident's daily activity is carried out in the immediate

company of other residents, all the daily activities are tightly scheduled and imposed from above, and various "enforced activities" bring the residents together to "fulfill the official aims of the institution."

30. For a more extensive discussion of the kinds of institutions that will be necessary to provide intermediate-level care, see my book: *Choosing Medical Care in Old Age: What Kind, How Much, When to Stop* (Cambridge, Mass.: Harvard University Press, 1994).

31. As of 1990, only 36 percent of internal-medicine residency programs included a formal curriculum in geriatrics. Among the programs that did have a curriculum, only 61 percent required their residents (physicians specializing in internal medicine) to participate. In 1993, the Institute of Medicine recommended that all residencies in internal medicine and family practice have six months of required geriatrics training by 1996 and nine months (out of three years) by 1999. This has not been widely instituted. See L. Chang, "The Geriatric Imperative: Meeting the Need for Physicians Trained in Geriatric Medicine," *Journal of the American Medical Association* 279 (1998): 1936–7.

32. J. Lynn, M. O'Connor, J. Dulac et al., "MediCaring: Development and Test Marketing of a Supportive Care Benefit for Older People," *Journal of the American Geriatrics Society* 47 (1999): 1058–64.

33. T. Fried, C. van Doorn, J. O'Leary et al., "Older Persons' Preferences for Site of Terminal Care," *Annals of Internal Medicine* 131 (1999): 109–12.

34. Projections of disability rates and nursing home residency rates are approximate. Current predictions, including upper and lower bounds, are available at the Administration on Aging Web site: www.aoa.dhhs.gov

35. See R. Binstock, "Changing Criteria in Old Age Programs: The Introduction of Economic Status and Need for Services," in *The Gerontologist,* 34 (1994): 726–30.

36. William Butler Yeats, "Sailing to Byzantium." Quoted in M. Rosenthal, ed., *Selected Poems and Two Plays by William Butler Yeats* (New York: Macmillan, 1962), 95. The full verse:

An aged man is but a paltry thing,
A tattered coat upon a stick, unless
Soul clap its hands and sing, and louder sing
For every tatter in its mortal dress,
Nor is there singing school but studying
Monuments of its own magnificence;
And therefore I have sailed the seas and come
To the holy city of Byzantium.

ACKNOWLEDGMENTS

It is my expectation that if the people on whose lives my stories are built read this book, their first reaction will be: But that didn't happen! My hope is that they will then say: But it could have happened! In short, I have felt free to embellish, to invent, and to graft stories from the lives of others onto the tales of the four people who are at the heart of this book. My additions and modifications were made for both didactic and artistic reasons: to give a comprehensive picture of frailty, and to create a compelling portrait of the protagonists. Two of the characters in the book are based on patients of mine who are very much alive, and who agreed to be interviewed for the book. They generously shared their reminiscences and reflections with me, understanding that I would build my characters around them. They understood that some of what they told me would not be included, or would be altered. They also understood that things would "happen to them" that never actually occurred, but they were nonetheless eager to have their experiences incorporated into the book.

One of the characters is based on a former patient who died before I conceived the idea for this book. Her daughter agreed to supplement my recollections and to tell me about her mother's past. She devoted many hours to remembering and interpreting her mother's life, particularly after the onset of frailty. Her daughter was familiar with my earlier books, and understood that although I planned to stick more closely to the actual events of her mother's life than I had previously, I would adapt the story.

The fourth character was never my patient, but was, as described, the father of an old friend. Since the family's response to frailty is a critical aspect of facing frailty, I thought it would be useful for one of the narratives to be related almost exclusively through the family's eyes. My friend recognized that this particular story would be mainly her version—but filtered through my memories of our earlier conversations. She let me interview her to refresh my memory on various points, to fill in some of the blanks in her father's history, and to think back on what dealing with chronic illness had been like for her.

One of the questions I struggled to answer in writing this book is how frail people find meaning in their lives. Their children are grown, they are retired—whether from homemaking or paying jobs—and they are seldom able to immerse themselves in hobbies, let alone new careers, because of their frailty. What sustains them? How do they cope in a society that tends to devalue them? Their answers are varied, and form part of their stories. The importance of family, and, more generally, of human relationships, is a recurring theme. For some, religion is a means of maintaining spiritual integrity in the face of physical decline. I would like to think that for the four people I interviewed—two daughters and two patients—this project contributed in a small way to creating a sense of meaning. My two patients saw the book as a way for them to reach out to others, through me as an intermediary, by helping those others both to accept and to transcend frailty. The two daughters saw the book as a memorial to their parents, a way for those often painful times to take on significance even after death. They recognize that this memorial is a meditation on their lives, not a biography.

Family and friends proved to be critically important for all four of the people whose stories I tell here; it was equally important for the author. My husband, Larry, dealt calmly and effectively with the many crises of self-confidence that punctuated the writing of this book. My sons, Daniel, Jeremy, and Jonathan, encouraged me to keep on writing stories. My parents, Ilse and Hans Garfunkel, with their vigor and excellent health, served as constant reminders that not everyone develops frailty. Jill Grinberg, my agent, had the wisdom, despite her youth, to agree that many baby boomers do not want to think about frailty, and to recognize that it is a tremendously important issue for all Americans to face. My editor, Angela von der Lippe, aided and abetted my first book, *Choosing Medical Care in Old Age* (Cambridge, Mass.: Harvard University Press, 1994), and encouraged me to submit a proposal for another book when she moved to Norton. Finally, those friends and colleagues who read parts of *Lifelines* in various incarnations provided me with invaluable feedback: Anne Fabiny, Gwen Frankfeldt, Susan Kalish, Karen Schoelles, and Valya Shapiro.